Promoting Health Through Creativity

I dedicate this book to the memory of my mother
Mollie Tubman Eichholzer
who encouraged me to open my eyes
to the realms beyond the material world

Promoting Health Through Creativity

For professionals in health, arts and education

Edited by

THERESE SCHMID

School of Health Sciences,
University of Newcastle, Australia

W
WHURR PUBLISHERS
LONDON AND PHILADELPHIA

© 2005 Whurr Publishers Ltd
First published 2005
by Whurr Publishers Ltd
19b Compton Terrace
London N1 2UN England and
325 Chestnut Street, Philadelphia PA 19106 USA

British Library Cataloguing in Publication Data

A catalogue record for this book
is available from the British Library.

ISBN 1 86156 478 3

Typeset by Adrian McLaughlin, a@microguides.net

Contents

Contributors

Editor

Therese Schmid MHlthSc(OT), AATR, DipOTNSW
Therese Schmid is a lecturer in occupational therapy at the School of Health Sciences, Faculty of Health, University of Newcastle, NSW, Australia. She has had extensive experience working in the field of mental health, in a therapeutic community, in community development programmes and in occupational therapy positions. Therese has published articles on experiential teaching and creativity.

Contributors

Estelle B. Breines PhD, OTR, FAOTA
Professor Estelle Breines holds the position of Chair, Department of Occupational Therapy Program at Seton Hall, New Jersey, America. Estelle obtained her BS in Occupational Therapy from New York University, her MA in Education and Behavioral Sciences from Kean University and her PhD in Occupational Therapy from New York University. She is President of the New Jersey Occupational Therapy Association. She is the author of six books and numerous chapters and journal articles.

Jennifer Creek MSc, DipCOT, Postgraduate Diploma in Art Therapy
Jennifer Creek is a freelance occupational therapist, an art therapist, a research and development officer for the British Association of Occupational Therapists, and a well-known author in the occupational therapy and mental health fields. Jennifer is the editor of two books and numerous articles. She has worked in the fields of adult mental health, learning disabilities and occupational therapy education.

Sally Denshire MAppSc(OT), DipOT
Sally Denshire is a lecturer in the Occupational Therapy Program at the School of Community Health, Charles Sturt University, Albury, NSW, Australia. She has worked in youth health, mental health, childbirth education, area health and curative education. Sally established the Youth Arts Programme in 1984 and the Adolescent Health Groupwork Service in 1985 at the Royal Alexandra Hospital for Children, Sydney, Australia. She entered academia in 1995. Her current research is concerned with creativity-based approaches to education, research and professional practice, and with life-writing and the human-related professions.

Frances Reynolds PhD, BSc, Diploma in Psychological Counselling
Dr Frances Reynolds is a lecturer in the School of Occupational Therapy at Brunel University of London. Frances obtained her BSc and PhD in Psychology. She is an Associate Fellow of the British Psychological Society, a Chartered Health Psychologist, and has published several articles and a chapter on creative activity.

Foreword

What an absorbing experience it is to gaze on the *Mona Lisa* and marvel at a masterpiece. Many of us might contemplate just how such a creative mind came into being; the same might be said after being enthralled by a ballerina, enchanted by a symphony performance or mesmerized by an intense drama. Perhaps most of us would dismiss as fantasy that we might indeed possess creativity remotely approaching those we admire as having a 'gift'. Therese Schmid not only effectively challenges the concept that creativity is rare, she demonstrates in a scholarly manner the important role creativity has in health and well-being, in particular, mental health.

Joining with a number of exceptional researchers, Therese enthusiastically articulates the everyday importance of creativity in our lives. Furthermore, her advocacy for proactive policies, which promote creativity as a resource to enhance quality of life and life more abundant is totally convincing. And why shouldn't it be, for Therese writes as she lives, with conviction and zeal. Having the privilege of working alongside her in a psychiatric facility in the past, it is obvious that the seeds of this work have been germinating for a long time, and that they grow from genuine personal experience. Certainly, my own creativity began its unveiling then and was positively influenced by her and the creative environment of those times.

Although these writings give strong focus to the vital role that creativity can play in better health outcomes – and they should be read by all clinicians, both practising and in training – the value of focusing on individual creativity has a central role in all disciplines, and drives the unfolding nature of knowledge. One can only hope that policymakers and administrators also take time to read this volume and respond creatively.

Trevor Waring
Chancellor and Conjoint Professor of Psychology
The University of Newcastle, NSW, Australia

Preface

All my life I have expressed myself through my creativity and the arts, and never more so than when I was employed (1971–1981) in an innovative psychiatry facility, Shortland Clinic, the psychiatric ward of the Royal Newcastle Hospital, NSW, Australia. This facility was a hive of creative energy and was a leader in the practice of therapeutic community principles, based on humanistic group psychotherapy theory. Howard Johnson, the psychiatrist in charge of the facility, was the most creative man I have ever worked with, and to his credit the facility remained an innovative, client-centred service for about 30 years. That service cannot be praised enough. The staff were given many opportunities to explore and develop their creativity. Many ex-staff have continued to work creatively in other positions and fields of work. Many of them have related that being a part of the clinic was an important milestone in their lives. Throughout my life I have continued to develop and use my creativity and art skills. I have, over many years, organized various types of arts and creativity workshops in the community, or at the request of health professionals.

In assembling this book I am urging for the acceptance of the health values of creativity. I can see that people are locked into a stunningly rapid technological revolution that is much too fast for their evolution. I can see how the incidence of depression and mental ill-health could continue to increase rapidly, at great cost to sufferers and their communities. I believe that the cultivation of everyday creativity is part of the solution and that it will require long term planning and funding. I only hope that what I am saying here becomes sufficiently widespread, and that enough people will speak up and add their weight to this request for action.

Throughout the years I have taken great comfort from many people with whom I have discussed the values of creativity for health and well-being. They include academics, teachers, health workers, psychologists, social workers, community groups, patients, craft groups and friends. They all believe it is a self-evident truth. However, from my experience, only 'proof' will result in action being taken or in funding being applied to promoting those values.

Much of this book is devoted to 'proof' of one kind or another, whether it be supportive research, anecdotal confirmation, examination of beliefs or an examination of the nature of people. The response I expect is that this is not enough proof to make policymakers act, but I hope that it is enough to generate serious inquiry. For that reason, the book discusses where and why the research so far is limited, and what research must be done. I hope there will be stimulation for future researchers, and, most importantly, that policymakers will recognize the good reasons to fund new research and learning programmes.

May you find it stimulating.

Therese Schmid
Maitland, NSW, Australia
March 2005

Acknowledgements

We are our history. Many special people in my history influenced my work, and travelled with me, on the quest for creativity. I am particularly grateful to Barry Pitman, who has been the 'plain English' editor. He has been able to cut to the chase with so many of my expressions and arguments, and has never failed in his support during the past two years. To Marian May, my dear friend and proofreader, a special thank you. It is a delight to add another chapter to our long friendship! Ann Wilcock, a well-known pioneer of occupational science and a friend of many years, suggested that I write the book. Thank you for your guidance through the inevitable difficulties. You warned that it would take many times longer than I expected. How right you were. To Paule Gauquie, Olwen Steel, Karen Murphy, Jan Callinan, Bill and Shirley Lennox, friends in Albury and Maitland, thank you for your endearing and enduring support. To my many colleagues at the University of Newcastle, especially within the School of Health Sciences, thank you for your encouragement. In addition, I am grateful to the time made available to me by the University of Newcastle, NSW, Australia. A special thank you to the chapter contributors, Estelle, Sally, Frances and Jennifer, for believing in me and giving much of their precious time. To all those individuals and group leaders who contributed to Chapters 7 and 9, it is your efforts that make the book sing. Thank you!

CHAPTER 1

Promoting health through creativity: an introduction

THERESE SCHMID

Background

Creativity plays a significant role in health and well-being. You will discover in these pages how essential, helpful, wonderful and exciting creativity can be in the quest for health. This chapter will introduce the overall concept and outline how the succeeding ones will provide evidence to support the argument of the book. Evidence will be offered from many areas of research and practice. Understanding and respecting the nature of creativity will open up many new possibilities for health professionals, health policymakers and educators.

The health industry and health promotion policymakers are in a unique position to promote this so-far-neglected factor of health to the general population, as well as towards vulnerable groups who are at risk of developing or suffering a mental illness. The outcomes would be improved public health, greater productivity and a reduced financial burden. Educators are in the unique position of enabling and encouraging every individual within the whole population to activate this health-and-pleasure-giving facet of their own nature.

This introductory chapter provides an overview of the relationship between 'health and well-being' and 'creativity'. Creativity will be defined and described. An examination of past research and of terminology (health, ill-health, occupation for health, health promotion, mental health, mental ill-health, mental well-being) will start to reveal some of the possibilities, some of the limitations and some of the difficulties. Forces operating against creativity will be identified, for this ground needs to be cleared before creativity is accepted on the health and the health promotion agenda. Further, it is argued that the outcomes of creativity are the very factors that are described in the literature as contributing to health and well-being. The contemporary population health model will then be described, for it is proposed that creativity for health can be incorporated into this model.

1

The book responds to the groundswell of interest in using 'creative activities' by a variety of health professionals, arts-in-health workers and creative arts therapists (music, art, dance and movement, drama). The population healthcare model is offered as a new perspective from which creativity for health and well-being can be promoted through health professionals and health promoters to all people, regardless of illness or disability. An active response to this could deliver creative opportunities to enhance health and well-being for people who have serious health difficulties; for example, youth who are at risk, those who are marginalized by a serious mental illness, the healthy aged and those who have a disability and are not able to access mainstream services. However, this is not a book about using creative activities in 'therapy', but rather it is a book about promoting creativity for the health and well-being of all people.

The writing of this book was also prompted by recent alarming statistics. It is estimated that, globally, by the year 2020, depression will be the leading cause of disability and the second-highest cause of the global burden of disease (WHO, 2002a). Mental and neurological disorders accounted for 12% of the total burden of disease worldwide, and it is estimated that this will increase to 15% by 2020 (WHO, 2001a). In Australia, mental disorders are the leading cause of disability burden, and depression is the leading cause of the non-fatal disease burden (Mathers et al., 1999; NSW Department of Health, 2002). The prevalence of depression increases with age, and depressive disorder is common among the elderly (WHO, 2001a). Worldwide, there are about 600 million people aged 60 and over, and by 2050 there will be two billion (WHO, 2002b). Compare these figures with world population figures. According to the United Nations (2002), the world's population is about 6.2 billion people, and it increases by 77 million a year. It is projected that by 2050 there will be 8.9 billion. Today, about two-thirds of all older people are living in the developing world; by 2025, it will be 75%. In the developed world, the very old (age 80+) is the fastest-growing population group (WHO, 2002b). An Australian non-governmental organization that works with the problems of depression states, 'depression and anxiety are the most common mental health problems in young people, affecting approximately 10% of children and up to 20% of adolescents in any one year' (beyondblue, 2001, p. 6).

Such statistics are challenging because, as will be shown, creativity deprivation can lead to depression. Much depends on how creativity is perceived by health policymakers, arts in health policymakers, health professionals, educationalists, the general population, the elderly, those who are at risk of developing a mental illness and those who have a mental illness.

Although there are volumes of literature on creativity, and the relationship between creativity and health is not new, there is scant literature that links this relationship to primary healthcare, the new public healthcare or health promotion. This deficiency will be discussed and proposals will be made.

A wealth of literature has been written on the therapeutic benefits of creative arts activities. Contributors have included: Azima and Azima (1957, 1959); Fidler and Fidler (1963); Rhyne (1970); Bissell and Mailloux (1981); Feder and Feder (1981); Landgarten (1981); Kielhofner (1983); Liebmann (1986); Reed (1986); Kaplan (1988); Dickerson and Kaplan (1991); Finlay (1993); Leary (1994); Breines (1995); Denshire (1996); Phillips (1996); Thompson and Blair (1998); Drake (1999); Fidler and Velde (1999); Levine and Levine (1999); Lloyd and Papas (1999), Atkinson and Wells (2000); Perrin (2001); Wilcock (2001); Creek (2002). For years, within mental healthcare settings, psychiatrists, occupational therapists, psychologists, social workers, other health professionals and arts therapists have used crafts, art, music, dance and drama as therapeutic agents in the clinical treatment of clients. Creativity has been implied within 'creative arts activities' but mostly it is not explicated as a vital process that, of itself, can be harnessed and applied to many of life's activities and occupations. Although professionals and policymakers are aware of the value of creative activities in therapy, they do not seem to be promoting the part that creativity can play in maintaining health and well-being and in preventing ill-health. Thus its full enabling powerful nature has not been called upon.

Although little research supports the notion that individual and community expressions of creativity are a vital part of health and well-being, all around us implicit messages commend creativity as healthy for everybody. For example, numerous kinds of community arts and craft guilds provide for this community expression. Governments and charities subsidize the expression of creativity in the organization of public and community arts festivals. People delight in their creative activities. Reviewing the literature will highlight the importance of these activities in their relationship to health and well-being. Further research is needed, particularly in the area of active community participation.

There is a particular difficulty in discussing 'creative activities'. People who take part in them experience joy and satisfaction, but when asked to describe 'creativity', they describe their experience as 'new', or 'innovative', or 'the idea came from nowhere', or 'doing craft is creative', or any number of attempts at description, but they cannot really find effective common words with which to answer the question. It seems the answer lies in the fact that creative activities are divided into parts. One part is the creative idea that makes the activity special or even unique to that individual or group. The other part is the expression of that idea. To be able to study creativity and learn to call on creativity it is important to have a language. This may also be a future subject of research.

Business managers and educationalists have, for many years, designed employee training courses in creative thinking and innovation (Gordon, 1961; Isaksen et al., 1993; Parnes, 1999; West and Rickards, 1999). The topic of creativity and innovation in relation to productivity has generated a lot of interest and research within a variety of disciplines (sociology, economics, organizational management, psychology). These disciplines embrace the notion that creativity can be learnt and can be a powerful tool in productivity. West and Rickards (1999, p. 55) envisaged that, 'In the 21st century world of electronically connected organizations, everyone will have a part to play as the creator and implementer of new ideas'. In this respect, creativity is not relegated to a special group of people, for example, the creative genius or top management. It should be recognized that such an extension in creative activity can apply even further into everybody's everyday world.

Although public education supports the value of teaching and learning the value of creativity, it is usually relegated to the optional arts subjects. Thus, creative thinking and the creative process are, more often than not, implied within subjects rather than explicated. It is not provided as a subject in its own right. If its connection is made only with the arts, then it depletes the significance of the role that creativity can play in everyday activities and occupations. Once creativity is demystified, students understand that there is a deep human need for creativity and that it has strong connections with health and well-being through self-esteem. They then feel more empowered and innovative every day throughout their lives. There is a wealth of educational research on this topic; however, the place of creativity within public education appears underdeveloped (Kneller, 1965; Edwards, 1986; Cropley, 1999a) and disconnected from its relationship with health.

Terminology

Promoting health and well-being through creativity is a challenging task. There are huge gaps in the literature, and confusion in terminology reigns throughout the whole spectrum of health and illness (well-being, mental health, mental ill-health, mental illness), and throughout understandings of creativity (creative thinking, innovation, creative activities, creativity in therapy, creative arts therapies – art, music, drama, dance therapy). To compound this topic, the field of health promotion introduces new terminology: health prevention, health education. In order to move forward through this labyrinth, it is necessary to define and describe these terms. Often, traditional vocabulary is not sufficient. New terms will be introduced in this book, and the reader is asked to consider how the new terms could avoid confusion. An example of the confusion is talking about the management of 'mental health' when what is meant is the management of 'mental illness'.

Definition of creativity

In this book the definition of creativity is based on the fundamental assumption that all people are creative or have the potential to be creative (Maslow, 1962, 1971, 1987; Rogers, 1970). Later in this chapter, and in Chapter 2, it will be established that the innate capacity to be creative is a biological reality. Creative thinking and behaviour exist to a greater or lesser degree in everyone. Some people have highly developed creative capacities. They may be involved in the arts, or in occupations such as architecture, design, teaching, science, advertising or research. Some people do not call upon their creativity, either because of the nature of their work, or their attitude to work, or because they do not know how to, or because they have not experienced the benefits of being creative.

The notion that creativity is connected to everyday activities, and therefore can be expressed through all activities, is included within the definition below. The terms 'everyday creativity' and 'ordinary creativity' were adopted by authors Ripple (1989) and Runco and Richards (1997) and Hasselkus (2002). Opportunities to be creative may be found in every kind of day-to-day activity, whether at work, home or in leisure; for example, in raising children, getting dressed for the day, doing community service, being involved in creative arts or crafts, drawing, painting, doing home repairs, instigating a new project at work, helping a friend problem solve, or dancing. Creativity can be everywhere. It results in the multitude of innovative changes that are at the heart of the evolution of ideas. The word *innovate* is defined in the *Concise Oxford Dictionary* (Pearsall, 1999) as 'make changes in something already existing, as by introducing new methods, ideas or products'. Such a change is an outcome from a creative process. It is an outcome that attains some level of adoption in the society or group under consideration (Lumsden, 1999). For example, it may mean the discovery of a new drug to cure a serious illness; it may be a new production process, or a new administrative method; it may be a family's new approach to decision-making. Creativity and innovation are regarded as interdependent activities, especially in change management (West and Rickards, 1999).

To date, creativity researchers generally identify the outcomes of creativity as products, ideas or behaviour (Richards, 1999). But also important are those positive feelings elicited by the expression of the inner-self (Csikszentmihalyi, 1996; Cropley, 1999b; Hirt, 1999; Russ,

1999). Findings from split-brain research on hemispheric exchange have revealed that appropriate affective states enable the hemispheric exchange necessary for creativity (Bogen and Bogen, 1999). Affective states are, therefore, included within this definition as a component and outcome of creativity. This is expanded in Chapter 2.

Creativity also refers to the 'creative process' that underlies the outcome; that is, the actual 'doing' of the creative activity (Kneller, 1965; Edwards, 1986; Cropley, 1999a). The creative process has been traditionally described as having progressive linear and sequential stages, which are information, saturation, incubation, illumination and verification (Edwards, 1986; Bogen and Bogen, 1999). However, more recently, Schuldberg (1999) has applied non-linear dynamical systems theory (chaos theory) to the creative process and products. The creative process includes those mental abilities and practical actions by which the creator intentionally goes beyond his or her prior experience to a new and meaningful outcome (Getzels and Csikszentmihalyi, 1976; Lumsden, 1999). Thus, being creative usually involves imaginative thought, general knowledge, and some mastery of the medium and the necessary skills. The creative process is seen as a process of discovery, which stimulates and guides expression by the creator, eliciting positive feelings and emotions, thereby promoting health and well-being. Therefore, for the purposes of this book, my following definition of creativity includes mental and affective factors, and the notion that creativity can be used in all activities.

> Creativity is the innate capacity to think and act in original ways, to be inventive, to be imaginative and to find new and original solutions to needs, problems and forms of expression. It can be used in all activities. Its processes and outcomes are meaningful to its user and generate positive feelings.

Health, ill-health and well-being

In the *Constitution of the World Health Organization* health was defined as 'a state of complete physical, mental and social well-being, and not merely the absence of disease or infirmity' (WHO, 1946, p. 2). Health writers frequently refer to this definition, for it has provided a basis for the current holistic view of health (Dowie et al., 1996; Tudor, 1996; Wilcock, 1998; AIHW, 2002).

Ill-health, as described by health promotional writers, is a negative quality of 'health' and includes disease, injury, dysfunction and illness within its description (Dowie et al., 1996; Tudor, 1996). However, these writers have furthered the notion that although people may have ill-health, that does not exclude them from having a sense of well-being. For example, a person with a degenerative disease may also think and feel that they have a comfortable and happy life.

Various health writers have subsequently built upon the 1946 World Health Organization definition. For example, the foundational definition of health in the Ottawa Charter for Health Promotion (WHO, 1986) and the subsequent definition of health promotion have firmly included the notions of individual, social and community empowerment, and these have formed the basis of community health and health promotion ever since.

The Ottawa Charter described health as 'a resource for everyday life, not the object of living. Health is a positive concept emphasising social and personal resources as well as physical capacities' (WHO, 1986, p. 1). Health promotion was defined as 'the process of enabling people to increase control over and to improve their health' (WHO, 1986, p. 1). A major goal of health promotion is to play a facilitating role in empowering people to balance their positive physical, mental and social health, by developing life skills and fostering self-esteem (Ashton and Seymour, 1991; Dowie et al., 1996; Tudor, 1996). Another goal is to prevent physical, mental and social ill-health.

Well-being is a concept that is less tangible than health and ill-health. Well-being is an old concept, and its connection to health has been made for centuries (Dowie et al., 1996; Wilcock, 1998). The description of well-being is generally subjective. For example, well-being is often described as feelings of pleasure, or various feelings of happiness, health and comfort, which can differ from person to person. An apt description of well-being is 'a subjective assessment of health which is less concerned with biological function than with feelings such as self-esteem and a sense of belonging through social integration' (Wilcock, 1998, p. 98). An outcome of creativity has often been described as an increase in self-esteem (Shaughnessy, 1987; Cropley, 1997; Hirt, 1999; Creek, 2002). This is relevant in that increasing self-esteem is a goal of health promotion. A 'sense of belonging' is often described by people after participating with others in doing creative activities, whether in leisure time or in paid employment activities (Finlay, 1993; Denshire, 1996), and again, is relevant to health promotion in that social health is another of its goals.

A current description of well-being from health promotion theorists is that well-being 'can be purely subjective, but to be a component of positive health it must arise from and reflect a process of empowerment, which may be enhanced through the development of life-skills' (Dowie et al., 1996, p. 26). This description, coupled with the World Health Organization (2001b) definition of mental well-being: 'a state in which the individual realizes his or her own abilities, can cope with the normal stresses of life, can work productively and fruitfully and is able to make a contribution to his or her community', has expanded the 1946 holistic definition of health enormously. It now reflects a sense of empowerment, autonomy and competence, and the ability to set and achieve goals. It now refers to emotions, thoughts and behaviours, and alludes to spiritual health (Wilcock, 1998). Thus, it is possible to interpret the definition as supporting a view that humans need to be engaged in a meaningful life in order to be healthy and have well-being.

The Australian indigenous notion of health and well-being (the Australian National Aboriginal Health Strategy, 1989, as cited in Commonwealth Department of Health and Aged Care, 2000a) reveals the importance of culture, the environment, harmony and interrelations to health and well-being. This will be expanded in Chapter 2.

Creativity, occupation and health

Definitions are not regarded as an absolute concept, but as something that can and must be constantly improved (Dowie et al., 1996; Tudor, 1996; Baum, 1998). In order to progress with the acceptance of creativity within the definition of health, an occupational perspective on health is included because creativity is critically linked to occupation (all activities).

An occupational perspective is one that theorizes that occupation is the natural biological mechanism for health and well-being (Wilcock, 1998, 2001). In this context 'occupation is everything that people do to occupy themselves' (Canadian Association of Occupational Therapists, 1997, p. 34). Moreover, Wilcock (1998) linked well-being to the engagement in occupation. One part of her research described an outcome in which a significant number of participants identified some form of occupational situation as one of the circumstances associated with their experience of well-being. From an occupational perspective of health, mental well-being 'embraces the belief that the potential range of individuals' occupations will allow each of them to be creative and adventurous as they experience all human emotions, explore and adapt appropriately, and without undue disruption meet their needs' (Wilcock, 1998, p. 103). It is implicit in this statement that creativity sits within daily life in a myriad of activities and occupations.

Overview of research

Creativity scholars and researchers have long examined the psychological bases of creativity, for example, the thinking processes, personality, motivation, the unconscious and inner drives, to name a few (Runco and Pritzker, 1999; Sternberg, 1999). Recent biological, neurological and psychological research has provided evidence that pathways exist for the expression of creativity (Myers, 1982; Vessels, 1982; Edwards, 1986; Hoppe and Kyle, 1990; Bogen and Bogen, 1999; Runco and Pritzker, 1999; see also Chapter 2). However, the link between creativity and health has mostly been implied. This kind of creativity research has been mostly reductionist in its aims, and quantitative in its methodology.

By contrast, humanistic theorists and researchers have been strong proponents in linking creativity to psychological health (Maslow, 1962; Rogers, 1970; Zinker, 1977). In humanistic theory, creativity and health are viewed as being directly connected to the notion of 'man's tendency to actualize himself, to become his potentialities' (Rogers, 1970, p. 140). This is now commonly termed 'self-actualization'. In his seminal 1954 paper, *Towards a Theory of Creativity* (Rogers, 1970), Rogers (an American psychologist and professor) provided a philosophy for creativity. In this paper Rogers paved the way towards the recognition of the creative potential in all people. He identified certain inner and external conditions that were necessary for creativity to flourish. The inner conditions included openness to experience and ability to respond to things as they are rather than through conventional categories, an internal locus of evaluation and the ability to toy with elements and concepts. The external conditions that Rogers described foster and nourish these inner conditions: psychological safety; accepting the individual as of unconditional worth; providing a climate in which external evaluation is absent; understanding empathically; and psychological freedom. Maslow, an American psychologist, in postulating about creativity, identified two kinds of creative behaviour: one as 'a special talent creativeness' and the other as 'self-actualizing creativeness' (Maslow, 1962, p. 37). He attributed the latter to a person who has a sound and integrated personality: a healthy person. Maslow described creativeness within self-actualizing people as 'a more widespread kind of creativeness which is the universal heritage of every human being that is born' (Maslow, 1962, p. 135) and 'which showed itself widely in the ordinary affairs of life' (Maslow, 1962, p. 137).

Recent studies that have investigated creativity, self-actualization and coping skills found that self-actualizing creative individuals seem to have effective coping skills (Runco et al., 1991; Sheldon, 1995). In particular, Sheldon's research suggested that the ability to tolerate conflict is a core characteristic of creative people, implying that this ability contributes to health and well-being. Research by Reynolds (2000), qualitative in design, explored women's views about the personal meanings of creative arts activities and the subjective part they played in the self-management of depression. The results of this research found that participants were inventive about coping skills, and that creative activities provided a safe haven in a stressful world, relaxation, shared interests and bonds with others, as well as a stronger sense of mastery – all of which serve as substantial resources to challenge depression. The implication of these findings is expanded in Chapter 2 and in Chapter 5.

Over the last 20 years there has been a growing interest by various health professionals and artists in using creativity therapeutically in general hospitals, in mental illness settings and in the community. The number of creative arts therapy educational programmes in Australia has increased. This book responds to this groundswell of interest. Humanistic theory and approaches are part of the philosophical belief systems and training of many health professionals, creative arts therapists (art, music, dance and movement, drama therapists), occupational therapists, social workers and clinical psychologists who use creative activities in therapy (Rhyne, 1970, 1973; Feder and Feder, 1981; Rubins, 1987; Finlay, 1993; Gilroy and Lee, 1995; McNiff, 1998; Atkinson and Wells, 2000; Creek, 2002). Part of that philosophical belief is that creativity positively contributes to the 'on-going growth, personal development and transcendence' of the individual (Richards, 1999, p. 684). This implies a positive bearing on health and well-being. Research designs and methodologies used by this group of health professionals are usually qualitative in design, and they often seek client perspectives and outcomes of creative activity in therapy. Despite this group's belief in self-actualization and creativity, the practice of creativity and creativity research within the health industry has remained mostly within a medical-illness perspective rather than within a health and wellness model. There is an upside to this. It is through the descriptions of the effectiveness of creative activities within therapy that the value of creativity in health and well-being for all has been identified. In Chapter 4, Jennifer Creek expands on these notions.

An emerging area of creativity research, termed 'everyday creativity research', views creativity as a survival capacity which allows all humans to adapt to changing environments, and therefore links creativity to evolution and hence to health and well-being (Lumsden, 1999; Richards, 1999). These notions will be expanded in the second chapter, where a theory of creativity is proposed.

Although some literature describes the importance of creative problem-solving in therapy, it is limited in describing the effect on health and well-being. Health professionals often refer to therapy as a creative process (Christiansen and Baum, 1997). However, on the whole, this notion is not explained. An exception to this is in the writings of American psychologist Joseph Zinker (1977). Zinker believed that there is an interconnection between creativity and psychology at a fundamental level. This fundamental level is the process of clients making changes in their behaviour, feelings and cognition. Zinker referred to this level as 'transformation, metamorphosis, change' (Zinker, 1977, p. 5). Also in his book is a very pertinent piece, where Laura Perls described therapy as being 'an ongoing creative adjustment to the potential in the therapeutic situation which includes therapist, clients and their developing relationship' (Zinker, 1977, dustjacket). Overall, this potential area of creativity research appears underdeveloped.

For decades, many creativity researchers and scholars have drawn attention to the notion that humans are estranged from their creativity, and that the mental well-being of many people is in jeopardy as a result (Barron, 1963; Kneller, 1965; Rogers, 1970; Shaughnessy, 1987; Richards, 1999; Runco and Pritzker, 1999). It is suggested that the alarming global increase in mental and neurological disorders may reflect this estrangement. Richards (1999) stated that a complex solution is required, which will enable the society to value creativity. It is intended that this book will be used as a resource from which can be formulated ideas and strategies that recognize the positive impact of creativity on health and well-being.

Creativity researchers and health researchers investigate many of the same psychological elements, such as personality, motivation, the unconscious, inner drives, cognition, moods and behaviour. The links between creativity research and health research appear to be clear and profoundly significant. The outcomes of creativity research indicate that creativity plays a major role in health and demands a central position in the promotion of health and mental well-being.

Current action

The Australian Commonwealth and State governments have responded to research and statistics by becoming proactive in improving intervention for mental illness and in reducing the disease burden at both population and individual levels (Raphael, 2000). For example, the Commonwealth and State governments have designated mental health as one of the five national health priority areas (Mathers et al., 1999). The population health model is currently being applied in the Australian public mental health industry, resulting in new policies and practices (Commonwealth Department of Health and Aged Care, 2000a, 2000b; Raphael, 2000). As an outcome, various initiatives are addressing these problems, for example, in the treatment of young adolescents with psychosis and those who are at risk of developing a mental illness (NSW Department of Health, 2002). beyondblue (2001), a non-government body, receives funding to provide preventive mental health interventions.

The Australia Council for the Arts and the Victorian Health Promotion Foundation, in particular, fund some preventive services for people who are at risk of developing a mental illness. These services do offer clients opportunities to be creative.

It is assumed in this book that health promotion policy incorporates a responsibility to empower the general population by providing knowledge of what constitutes a healthy life, as described by Dowie et al. (1996) and Tudor (1996). However, as yet, there is little funding directed to promotions designed to educate the general public about the connections between 'creativity' and 'health and well-being'.

Ageing and creativity

In addition to the alarming statistics in the increase of mental disorders, both the mortality and fertility rates are decreasing across the globe, resulting in higher life expectancies and an ageing population (Mathers et al., 1999). Just as the population of Australia is ageing, so it is for the UK, America, Canada and many other countries. The implications for health promotion are likely to be dramatic, with an increasing cost burden on social security and healthcare.

Glass et al. (1999) conducted a prospective cohort study with annual mortality follow-up over 13 years, with a random sample of 2761 men and women aged 65 and older. They examined any association between social, productive or physical activity, and mortality. This research concluded that social and productive activities that involve little or no enhancement of fitness lower the risk of all-cause mortality as much as fitness activities do. It validated an occupational perspective on health, that doing activities or occupations enhances health and well-being. This research omitted to consider whether creativity was a part of the activities and whether it affected mortality. However, creativity research is revealing not only how ageing influences creativity, but also that creativity influences ageing and longevity (Dawson and Baller, 1972; Australian Pensioners' and Superannuants' Federation, 1995; Fisher and Specht, 1999; Levy and Langer, 1999).

As people live longer, the demand for opportunity for activities in numerous areas of life will be unprecedented. Although health policy acknowledges the increase in the numbers of elderly people, support or funding is limited for the infrastructure for those social and productive activities that will keep elderly people healthy, contributing to the society, out of hospitals and in their own homes. Support or funding to develop the creative opportunities inherent in those activities and make them even more valuable, is very little.

Health policy does fund senior citizens' groups. Substantial funds are in place to provide creative arts entertainment to all age groups. Health services in the form of home care are provided to help keep people in their homes. Superannuation incentives are provided for those who choose to work beyond retiring age. But, where is the promotion and support for the creative capacities that might expose new ideas and innovations that could be of value to the community, and personally reward the creative person with a boost in satisfaction and self-esteem? These are the seeds of good health and well-being. Such creativity is in all people, but mostly latent. All people need to learn how to access it, and they can, if the supporting processes are available. To date, those processes, which include education, are almost totally ignored. There are exceptions. One of the most outstanding is the 'Performing Older Women's Circus' funded by VicHealth, the Government health body in Victoria, Australia, which aims to promote healthy exercise. Participants, however, claim that exercise is only part of the gain. They claim an exciting and stimulating feeling as a result of the shared act of creating new ideas for their activities, and they say that this gives them feelings of self-esteem and well-being. This will be referred to later in Chapter 7.

Funding

The Australian total health expenditure for 1999–2000 was $53.7 billion (AIHW, 2002). Depression, including suicide and self-inflicted injury, accounts for 4.9% of that burden, making it the third leading cause of burden of disease in Australia (Mathers et al., 1999). That represents $2.63 billion. If 'creativity' could relieve the cost burden of depression by just 10%, it would be worth a very large investment in education, promotion and community funding to bring it about. As an investment in health, it could not be wasted. As an investment in people, it could have stunning and unprecedented results in 'health and well-being', in the enjoyment and satisfaction in life at all ages, and in innovation and productivity. This potential could only be to the advantage of all people in all countries.

The health cost of depression is not the only loss to the community that could be reduced substantially through creativity. There are indirect costs. There may be loss through co-morbidity. There is an enormous loss through days not worked, or through sick leave. There is an enormous loss of productivity through 'feeling depressed', boredom or disenchantment. There is a loss through skills withdrawn because of disillusionment. There is a loss of the opportunistic gain that could be won from creative innovations by individuals or groups. Investment in individual creativity could pay big dividends.

Forces operating against creativity in health promotion

In order for creativity to be accepted and placed on the agenda of health, and hence health promotion, the confusion in terminology needs to be resolved. Clear understanding needs to operate between all concerned health professionals and policymakers. The elements of creativity for positive health and well-being need to be clearly communicated and accepted. These elements need to be seen as being embedded within mental well-being. In particular, mental well-being needs to be viewed as a vital part of health for the whole population, not just for those who have a mental illness or those who are at risk of developing mental illness (Dowie et al., 1996; Tudor, 1996). However, the promotion of mental well-being is in its infancy (Trent, 1992; Dowie et al., 1996; Tudor, 1996). Tudor (1996) identified a number of factors that work against the promotion of mental well-being: a lack of public recognition and acceptance; inadequate knowledge of the system of conditions for mental health; insufficient material and personal resources; and little co-operation with the institutions, groups or persons participating in the process. If it is difficult to promote mental well-being on the health promotion agenda, it follows that it will also be difficult for creativity to be incorporated into the health promotion agenda.

Another huge obstacle to placing creativity on the health promotion agenda is the existing cultural belief that creativity belongs only to an élite. Health promotion would need to facilitate the demystification of creativity on numerous fronts.

This book is not about health promotion. It is about the inclusion of one element of health, creativity, in health promotion. It challenges the lack of understanding (and acceptance) of the value of creativity to health and well-being. It provides current material about creativity and health and well-being, and its various links to health promotion. It highlights the lack of collaboration between concerned groups and organizations and offers ways out of what Tudor (1996, p. 5) terms 'paradigm prisons'.

The modern definition of health is holistic in perspective; however, within the healthcare system and associated funding policy, health promotion is still largely based on a medical perspective, that is, from the point of view of the absence of disease, rather than what constitutes a healthy life (Dowie et al., 1996; Tudor, 1996; Wilcock, 1998). A medical perspective is vital in health promotion. However, a perspective must be included for maintaining health and well-being without the implication of disease, and that requires language that clearly describes the difference. Paradigm prisons therefore need to be identified. Collaboration between health, arts and education policymakers and the various arts-in-health workers and health professionals could, therefore, determine new directions for promotion.

Linking creativity, well-being and health for promotion

Lack of social support, lack of homeostasis (being in balance), significant life events that provoke a degree of unmanageable stress in individuals or communities, and lack of meaningful occupations will work against mental and social well-being.

Wilcock (1998) and Blair and Hume (2002) highlight the importance of social contact and social support networks as factors in well-being. Without social support and integration, people become ill. The emerging field of study, 'social health', also supports this notion (Baum, 1998). It was included in the 1946 World Health Organization definition of health and emerged in Australia in the 1980s. Group creative activities can satisfy some elements needed for health and well-being through social contact and interpersonal relationships. Many benefits of creative activities that are both therapeutic and desirable in everyday healthy life, such as self-esteem, coping, self-concept and identity, physical and cognitive processes, experiencing control, perceptual ability, new ways of communicating and insight, have been identified by health professionals (Azima and Azima, 1957, 1959; Borg and Bruce, 1991; Finlay, 1993; Drake, 1999; Creek, 2002). Sally Denshire explores these concepts further in Chapter 8.

The Concise Oxford Dictionary (Pearsall, 1999) defines homeostasis as 'the maintenance of a stable equilibrium, especially through physiological processes'. It is essential to human health. When either external or internal pressures disturb the balance, individuals tend to operate at a higher rate of energy and, as a consequence, block attention to any psychological or physiological distress. If the pressures continue, or if an individual does not have the capacity to respond positively to significant life events, then well-being will be diminished and the individual can be in danger of either physical or psychological ill-health (Blair and Hume, 2002). If there was a general acceptance and recognition of the health value of being creative in everyday activities, and if supporting health-promotional materials were available for personal and community resources, there would be more chance for individual and for community homeostasis.

A basic belief of occupational therapists is that occupation brings meaning to life and 'that meaning of an occupation is individually and culturally determined' (Canadian Association of Occupational Therapists, 1997, p. 36). Without meaning in everyday occupations, people usually have a diminished sense of well-being. The health and well-being of an individual or a community is affected by any deprivation, alienation or imbalance in occupation or activities (Wilcock, 1998). An example of occupational deprivation is where the widespread problem of unemployment decreases the opportunity for people to engage in meaningful occupations. These people are vulnerable to psychological ill-health or depression.

Being mindful of the health value of being creative enables people to affect their own health. It provides them with a choice about incorporating creativity within their lives. In turn, people who include creativity in their daily lives improve their health and reduce the 'disability burden' (Mathers et al., 1999). Creativity elicits feelings of worth, self-esteem, satisfaction, pride, interest, curiosity, excitement, hope and elation. These are some of the psychological elements involved in achieving a creative outcome (Cropley, 1999b). In addition, creativity engages cognitive processes that contribute to mental well-being, for example, perception, remembering, learning, convergent thinking, motivation, problem-finding, problem-solving, divergent thinking, openness, tolerance for ambiguity, willingness to take risks, evaluation of configurations for novelty, knowledge of the field, familiarity with norms and conventions, making results available to others, mastering of a form of communication, willingness to risk being laughed at, societal evaluation, effectiveness and relevance (Cropley, 1999b).

Part of the orientation of this book is concerned with governments being proactive about the mental well-being of the whole population. Tudor (1996), Wilcox (1998, 2001) and Blair and Hume (2002) have identified a range of strategies to promote mental well-being that can have positive effects on individuals and communities, for example encouraging the development of individual skills and resources, enhancing the socio-economic environment and promoting occupation for health. In particular, Tudor (1996) identified a number of elements that could be targeted for promotional or preventive action, for example autonomy, coping, tension and stress management, self-concept and identity, self-esteem, self-development, change, social support and involvement. These elements have long been identified as properties of normal personality development. Creative researchers have drawn attention to the similarities between these elements and those that are identified as characteristics of creative people (Cropley, 1990). Research has also demonstrated that the ability to tolerate conflict is a core characteristic of creative people and that people who are self-actualizing and creative seem to have effective coping skills (Runco et al., 1991; Sheldon, 1995). The connection is so strong that little argument can be made against the proposition that creativity is essential to health and well-being.

Population health model

'Population health' is a relatively new term that is replacing the term 'public health'. Since the 1980s, a new public health philosophy has emerged (Baum, 1998; Ashton and Seymour, 1991; Commonwealth Department of Health and Aged Care, 2000a). The term 'public health' is being replaced for two reasons: it is equated with publicly funded structures, and it is seen to be too limiting in that its central view is a medical model and hence does not include other health professionals' views of health (Ashton and Seymour, 1991). The 'population health' approach recognizes that health and illness, at a personal, local, national and global level, result from the complex interplay of biological, psychological, social, environmental and economic factors. A 'population health' approach attends to the health status and health needs of both whole populations and population groups. It encompasses population needs assessment, developing and implementing intervention, monitoring trends and evaluating outcomes (Commonwealth Department of Health and Aged Care, 2000a; Raphael, 2000).

Health promotion, prevention and early intervention activities

This 'population health' approach aims to utilize the model of a whole range of intervention from good health promotion to prevention, treatment and maintenance, and to identify how these can be applied at population and individual levels right across the life span.

Specifically, the 'population health' model provides an ideal conceptual framework for promoting mental well-being and preventing mental illness, by providing early intervention as well as standard treatment and maintenance (Commonwealth Department of Health and Aged Care, 2000a, 2000b). This model, using mental well-being as its focus, can very comfortably include creativity in its perspective.

At the prevention level, intervention is planned to occur before the onset of a disorder. There are three kinds of preventive intervention: universal, selective and indicated. Universal prevention is an intervention for whole populations, and its method is usually health education (Dowie et al., 1996). Typical examples are the encouragement of physical fitness, the encouragement of good diet, the promotion of anti-influenza injections, and media campaigns to reduce the stigma of mental illness.

Selective preventive intervention targets high-risk subgroups within a population. Examples are young people who are at increased risk of developing a mental illness or disorder, those who are vulnerable to depression (beyondblue, 2001) and schoolchildren in disadvantaged populations (Raphael, 2000).

Indicated preventive intervention is intervention aimed at groups and individuals who are at a very high risk of disorder onset (Raphael, 2000). For example, the Young People and Psychiatric Illness – Intervention and Assessment (YPPI-IA) based at the Central Coast Mental Health Service in NSW, Australia, is a service for those suffering from a first-episode psychosis.

Raphael (2000) emphasized that within the framework of the population health model there are possibilities to be proactive. This suggests that the promotion of mental well-being and creativity could be linked and therefore promoted right across the full range of intervention in population health.

A favourable characteristic of the population health model is that it recognizes and includes a broad range of stakeholders and partners (Raphael, 2000). For example, in the mental illness area, in addition to the public healthcare workers, it includes the wider community (GPs and the families of those with a mental illness), consumers and carers (consumer rights advocates are now paid workers on-site in psychiatric hospitals), informal support systems and networks (various self-help groups, the Schizophrenia Fellowship) and non-governmental organizations (the Psychiatric Rehabilitation Association, the Association of the Relatives and Friends of the Mentally Ill, beyondblue; to name a few). This enables a broad scope for intervention and satisfies the broader sociocultural and community aspects within the current definitions of health and health promotion.

In summary, the population health model in Australia has implemented preventive intervention. However, this has mostly been restricted to the selective or indicative level of care. For example, a range of media promotional strategies has been aimed at the general population to increase awareness of, and prevent, mental illness. The media campaigns were targeted to lessen the stigma of mental illness, and appear to have been successful. However, again, health promotion has been designed as an intervention from a medical perspective. Promoting mental well-being is not the same as promoting an understanding of mental illness. Promoting mental well-being and healthy methods of maintaining it must be supported by methods similar to promoting health through physical fitness or through healthy diet.

The model for promoting health and well-being through creativity

The population health approach, because it maintains a holistic view, embraces a variety of perspectives on health. This book argues that further perspectives on health need to be accepted. Wilcock (1998, 2001) has argued for an occupational perspective for health. It is argued here that creativity can be a recognizable part of all occupations or activities. If accepted, this would then support the concept that creativity should be an important part of health and well-being in health promotion policy and strategies. By accepting this, policymakers would then be in a position to promote creativity for health and well-being, through the population health model, for all members of the community, not only for those who have ill-health, a disability or a mental illness.

The universal, preventive-intervention level of the model would be the most valuable level at which the promotion of health and well-being through creativity could take place. Various 'creativity for health and well-being' education methods could be designed, ranging from media campaigns to education systems at all levels.

Current selective and indicated prevention interventions for mental illness within community settings and the mental-illness treatment and maintenance services within psychiatric settings do not, as yet, provide a sufficient range of creative activities for their clients. Some settings do provide a creative arts programme. Although commendable, they are few in number and are not necessarily linked to the population health model. Nevertheless, they are important examples of what could be multiplied in many different ways and at many different levels. Clients and providers must see creativity as a skill that can be learnt, enjoyed and applied to everyday activities, thereby increasing self-esteem and coping skills. Chapter 9 of this book will describe a range of services that are sponsored and funded by several stakeholders and partners, and which utilize creativity.

It is hoped that governments and policymakers will come to appreciate that funding health promotion and community services which promote creativity for health will, in the long run, not only save the Government money, but also increase health and well-being across the full spectrum of the population.

Plan of the book

The following chapters support the argument that has been set out in Chapter 1.

Chapter 2, by Therese Schmid, offers evidence that creativity is an innate human biological capacity. Literature from the 'new sciences': palaeoanthropology, cultural anthropology and evolutionary psychology, is married with occupational science, neuroscience and psychology. This synthesis offers creativity research a way forward in that creativity is placed within the capacity of all people, and in everyday activities. Therese Schmid attributes the burgeoning of creativity to the significant

changes in the 'modern human mind' that evolved during the Upper
Palaeolithic Period. She views creativity as a major driving force in the evolution of human nature, linked to health and well-being through the
pressure to adapt and survive. This material is drawn together in a discussion about the significant consequences of the waning of the demand
for, and the expression of, creativity in modern everyday activities. In con-
clusion, the challenge of the restoration of creativity is introduced. This is
discussed further in Chapter 10.

In Chapter 3, Professor Estelle Breines also focuses on evolution, but
views the connection between creativity and health and well-being
through the sociocultural evolution of creative activities. According to
Breines, creativity is built on two interrelated phenomena of performance
– the automatic and the deliberate – and is linked to human development.
Breines examines how, in the evolution of human beings, their natural
creativity in developing life's tasks and occupational choices serves as a
foundation for achieving and maintaining health. Professor Breines has
written extensively on notions of adaptation and occupational genesis.

In Chapter 4, Jennifer Creek highlights the therapeutic benefits of creativity by exploring the relationship between creativity and health. Creek
identifies groups of healthcare professionals, including occupational therapists, music therapists, drama therapists, dance and movement
therapists and art therapists, who use that relationship to inform their
therapeutic approaches. Four approaches to therapy using creative activities are described. Examples are given to illustrate how these approaches
have been used in clinical practice. One theme that runs through the
accounts is that the therapeutic use of creative arts is experienced as powerful yet safe and non-intrusive.

In chapters 5 and 6, Frances Reynolds examines creativity research
comprehensively, reviewing studies that connect creativity with health
and well-being. Chapter 5 considers studies that address the influences
which shape individual creativity. Reynolds' findings indicate gaps in
research on the origins of creativity, and on the everyday forms of creativity. She observes that studies on the assessment of creativity lack the
identification of the nurturing social influences which help people to fulfil their creative potential. She recommends the use of self-report and
phenomenological research methodologies, which would complement
the evidence gained from the quantifying methodologies used in most
creativity research.

In Chapter 6, Reynolds continues her rigorous examination of studies
that have explored the influence of creativity on physical and psychological well-being. She calls for further quantifying of changes in physical and
psychological functioning, and in the identification of the critical processes involved in creativity. She argues for a review of the definitions of

creativity and for studies of everyday forms of creativity. This examination offers positive directions for interdisciplinary dialogue and research.

For Chapter 7, Therese Schmid set out to gather personal expressions of how people felt about the effects that their creative activities had on their health and well-being. The responses were willing and unanimous. Some of the contributors have an illness, or have recovered from illness, and, for them, creativity has been transformational. For others, creativity is seen as one of the pleasures of life. This chapter offers a view of a range of experiences: the circus; working with fibre; knitting; writing; painting; gardening; song writing; and drawing. The accounts, gathered through invitation, are not intended to represent a research project. The aim of the chapter was to offer readers rich subjective narratives that link creativity to health and well-being, and to reveal some opportunities for research.

In Chapter 8, Sally Denshire discusses contemporary theories and issues concerning effective groupwork practice in using creative activities for health and well-being. She supports this with examples from her practice as an occupational therapist, from her experience as a community worker, and from her current lecturing position. Sally distinguishes the values of creativity-based groupwork and offers ways to integrate these into a health service.

For Chapter 9, Therese Schmid has gathered accounts from group leaders about a variety of successful projects that promote health, mental well-being and social and community well-being through a range of innovative arts or arts therapy programmes, or creative activity programmes. They include government-funded and non-government-funded programmes. This chapter is designed to augment the discussion in Chapter 8 about creativity-based groupwork. The members of the groups include the healthy, people in recovery, youth, the elderly and some with an enduring illness or disability. In all the accounts, the outcomes for health and well-being are positive and highly valued by the participants, and they demonstrate the increased benefits of doing creative activities in a group setting. The chapter is not intended to represent a research project, but, as for Chapter 7, useful consensual truth can be derived from it. The chapter may encourage readers to note opportunities for research. Some of the accounts describe evaluation tools and research methods. The programmes described are:

- 'Arts in Health' projects, Newcastle, Australia.
- The development of a creativity course at the University of Chile.
- 'Artsenta', New Zealand.
- 'SoundMinds', London, UK.
- 'Performing Older Women's Circus' and the 'Older Persons' Circus', NSW, Australia.
- 'Small Towns Big Picture – The Art of Engagement', Victoria, Australia.

- 'Bellbird Gardens', NSW, Australia.
- 'Wilderness Theatre', NSW, Australia.
- 'The Sculpture Trail' – Artnode, NSW, Australia.
- 'Material Women – Weaving Fabric and Stories', Western Australia.

In Chapter 10, key aspects of the book are summarized by Therese Schmid to reaffirm the values of creativity and the links between creativity and health and well-being. Therese emphasizes that the health problems being generated by rapid technological change demand new approaches. Long term strategies for health promotion, research, education and community involvement are suggested.

References

Ashton J, Seymour H. The New Public Health. The Liverpool Experience. Philadelphia, PA: Open University Press, 1991.

Atkinson K, Wells C. Creative Therapies. A Psychodynamic Approach within Occupational Therapy. Cheltenham: Stanley Thornes, 2000.

Australian Institute of Health and Welfare. Australia's Health (AIHW Cat. No. AUS-25). Canberra: Australian Government Publishing Service, 2002.

Australian Pensioners' and Superannuants' Federation. Older Australians and the Arts: A Report for the Australia Council. Redfern, NSW: Australia Council, 1995.

Azima H, Cramer-Azima F, Wittkower ED. Analytic group art therapy. International Journal of Group Psychotherapy 1957; 7: 243–60.

Azima H, Azima FJ. Projective group therapy. International Journal of Group Psychotherapy 1959; 9: 176–83.

Barron F. Creativity and Psychological Health. Princeton, NJ: Van Nostrand, 1963.

Baum F. The New Public Health. An Australian Perspective. Melbourne: Oxford University Press, 1998.

beyondblue. beyondblue bulletin, November, 2001. (Accessed November 2001 from www.beyondblue.org.au)

Bissell JC, Mailloux Z. The use of crafts in occupational therapy for the physically disabled. American Journal of Occupational Therapy 1981; 35: 369–74.

Blair SEE, Hume CA. Health, wellness and occupation. In: Creek J (ed.), Occupational Therapy and Mental Health (third edition). London: Churchill Livingstone, 2002; 15–27.

Bogen JE, Bogen GM. Split brains: interhemispheric exchange in creativity. In: Runco MA, Pritzker SR (eds), Encyclopedia of Creativity (Vol. 2). London: Academic Press, 1999; 571–5.

Borg B, Bruce MAG. The Group System. Thorofare, NJ: Slack, 1991.

Breines EB. Occupational Therapy. Activities from Clay to Computers. Theory and Practise. Philadelphia, PA: FA Davis, 1995.

Canadian Association of Occupational Therapists. Enabling Occupation. An Occupational Therapy Perspective. Ottawa: CAOT, 1997.

Christiansen C, Baum C (eds). Occupational Therapy: Enabling Function and Well-being (second edition). Thorofare, NJ: Slack, 1997.

Commonwealth Department of Health and Aged Care. Promotion, Prevention and Early Intervention for Mental Health – A Monograph (PN2787). Canberra: Commonweath Department of Health and Aged Care, Mental Health and Special Programs Branch, 2000a.

Commonwealth Department of Health and Aged Care. National Action Plan for Promotion, Prevention and Early Intervention for Mental Health 2000 (PN2786). Canberra: Commonwealth Department of Health and Aged Care, Mental Health and Special Programs Branch, 2000b.

Creek J (Ed.). Occupational Therapy and Mental Health (third edition). London: Churchill Livingstone, 2002.

Cropley AJ. Creativity and mental health in everyday health. Creativity Research Journal 1990; 3: 167–79.

Cropley AJ. Fostering creativity in the classroom: general principles. In: Runco MA (ed.), The Creativity Handbook. Cresskill NJ: Hampton Press, 1997; 83–114.

Cropley AJ. Education. In: Runco MA, Pritzker SR (eds), Encyclopedia of Creativity (Vol. 1). London: Academic Press, 1999a; 629–37.

Cropley AJ. Definitions of creativity. In: Runco MA, Pritzker SR (eds), Encyclopedia of Creativity (Vol. 1). London: Academic Press, 1999b; 511–24.

Csikszentmihalyi M. Creativity. Flow and the Psychology of Discovery and Invention. New York, NY: HarperCollins, 1996.

Dawson AM, Baller WR. Relationship between creative activity and the health of elderly persons. Journal of Psychology 1972; 82: 49–58.

Denshire S. A decade of creative occupation: the production of a youth arts archive in a hospital site. Journal of Occupational Science: Australia 1996; 3: 93–8.

Dickerson A, Kaplan SH. A comparison of craft use and academic preparation in craft modalities. American Journal of Occupational Therapy 1991; 45: 11–17.

Dowie RS, Tannahill C, Tannahill A. Health Promotion. Models and Values (second edition). Oxford: Oxford University Press, 1996.

Drake M. Crafts. Therapy and Rehabilitation. Thorofare, NJ: Slack, 1999.

Edwards B. Drawing On the Artist Within. How to Release Your Hidden Creativity. Glasgow: Fontana/Collins, 1986.

Feder E, Feder B. The Expressive Arts Therapies. Thorofare, NJ: Prentice-Hall, 1981.

Fidler G, Fidler J. Occupational Therapy – A Communication Process in Psychiatry. New York, NY: Macmillan, 1963.

Fidler GS, Velde BP. Activities: Reality and Symbol. Thorofare, NJ: Slack, 1999.

Finlay L. Groupwork in Occupational Therapy. London: Chapman & Hall, 1993.

Fisher BJ, Specht DK. Successful aging and creativity in later life. Journal of Aging Studies 1999; 13: 457.

Getzels JW, Csikszentmihalyi M. The Creative Vision: A Longitudinal Study of Problem Finding in Art. New York, NY: Wiley, 1976.

Gilroy A, Lee C. Art and Music Therapy and Research. New York, NY: Routledge, 1995.

Glass TA, de Leon CM, Marottoli RA, Berkman LF. Population based study of social and productive activities as predictors of survival among elderly Americans. British Medical Journal 1999; 319: 478–83.

Gordon WJJ. Synectics. The Development of Creative Capacity. New York, NY: Harper & Row, 1961.

Hasselkus BR. The Meaning of Everyday Occupation. Thorofare, NJ: Slack, 2002.

Hirt ER. Mood. In: Runco MA, Pritzker SR (eds), Encyclopedia of Creativity (Vol. 1). London: Academic Press, 1999; 241–50.

Hoppe KD, Kyle NL. Dual brain, creativity and health. Creativity Research Journal 1990; 3: 150–7.

Isaksen SC, Murdock MC, Firestien RL, Treffinger DJ. Nurturing and Developing Creativity: The Emergence of a Discipline. Thorofare, NJ: Ablex, 1993.

Kaplan KL. Directive Group Therapy. Thorofare, NJ: Slack, 1988.

Kielhofner G (ed.). Health Through Occupation – The Theory and Practise in Occupational Therapy. Philadelphia, PA: FA Davis, 1983.

Kneller GF. The Art and Science of Creativity. New York, NY: Holt, Reinhart & Winston, 1965.

Landgarten HB. Clinical Art Therapy. New York, NY: Brunner/Mazel, 1981.

Leary S. Activities for Personal Growth: A Comprehensive Handbook of Activities for Therapists. Sydney: Maclennan & Petty, 1994.

Levine SK, Levine EG (eds). Foundations of Expressive Arts Therapy. Theoretical and Clinical Perspectives. London: Jessica Kingsley, 1999.

Levy B, Langer E. Aging. In: Runco MA, Pritzker SR (eds), Encyclopedia of Creativity (Vol. 1). London: Academic Press, 1999; 45–52.

Liebmann M. Art Therapy for Groups. A Handbook of Themes, Games and Exercises. London: Routledge, 1986.

Lloyd C, Papas V. Art as therapy within occupational therapy in mental health settings: a review of the literature. British Journal of Occupational Therapy 1999; 62: 31–4.

Lumsden CJ. Evolving creative minds. Stories and mechanism. In: Sternberg J (ed.), The Handbook of Creativity. Cambridge: Cambridge University Press, 1999; 153–68.

McNiff S. Art-based Research. London: Jessica Kingsley, 1998.

Maslow AH. Toward a Psychology of Being. Princeton, NJ: Van Nostrand, 1962.

Maslow AH. The Farther Reaches of Human Nature. New York, NY: The Viking Press, 1971.

Maslow AH. Motivation and Personality (third edition). New York, NY: Harper & Row, 1987.

Mathers C, Vos T, Stevenson C. The Burden of Disease and Injury in Australia – Summary Report (AIHW Cat. No. PHE18). Canberra: Australian Institute of Health and Welfare, 1999.

Myers JT. Hemispheric research: an overview with some implications for problem solving. Journal of Creative Behaviour 1982; 16: 197–211.

NSW Department of Health. The Health of the People of New South Wales – Report of the Chief Health Officer. Sydney: Public Health Division, NSW Department of Health, 2002.

Parnes SJ. Programs and courses in creativity. In: Runco MA, Pritzker SR (eds), Encyclopedia of Creativity (Vol. 2). London: Academic Press, 1999; 465–77.

Pearsall J (ed.). The Concise Oxford Dictionary (10th edition). Oxford: Oxford University Press, 1999.

Perrin T. Don't despise the fluffy bunny: a reflection from practice. British Journal of Occupational Therapy 2001; 64: 129–34.

Phillips ME. The use of drama and puppetry in occupational therapy during the 1920s and 1930s. American Journal of Occupational Therapy 1996; 50: 229–33.

Raphael B. A Population Health Model for the Provision of Mental Health Care (Publication no. 2735). Canberra: AusInfo, 2000.

Reed KL. Tools of practice: heritage or baggage? American Journal of Occupational Therapy 1986; 40: 597–605.

Reynolds R. Managing depression through needlecraft creative activities: a qualitative study. The Arts in Psychotherapy 2000; 27: 107–14.

Rhyne J. The Gestalt art experience. In: Fagan J, Shepherd IL, Gestalt Therapy Now. New York, NY: Harper & Row, 1970; Chapter 22.

Rhyne J. The Gestalt Art Experience. Monterey, CA: Brooks/Cole, 1973.

Richards R. Everyday creativity. In: Runco MA, Pritzker SR (eds), Encyclopedia of Creativity (Vol.1). London: Academic Press, 1999; 683–9.

Ripple RE. Ordinary creativity. Contemporary Educational Psychology 1989; 14: 189–202.

Rogers CR. Toward a theory of creativity. In: Vernon PE (Ed.), Creativity: Selected Readings. Harmondsworth: Penguin, 1970; 137–51.

Rubins JA. Approaches to Art Therapy. Theory and Technique. New York, NY: Brunner/Mazel, 1987.

Runco MA, Ebersole P, Mraz W. Creativity and self-actualisation. Journal of Social Behaviour and Personality 1991; 6: 161–7.

Runco MA, Pritzker SR (eds). Encyclopedia of Creativity (vols 1 and 2). London: Academic Press, 1999.

Runco MA, Richards R (eds). Eminent Creativity, Everyday Creativity, and Health. London: Ablex, 1997.

Russ SW. Emotion/affect. In: Runco MA, Pritzker SR (eds), Encyclopedia of Creativity (Vol. 1). London: Academic Press, 1999; 659–68.

Schuldberg D. Chaos theory and creativity. In: Runco MA, Pritzker SR (eds), Encyclopedia of Creativity (Vol. 1). London: Academic Press, 1999; 259–72.

Shaughnessy MF. Health through creativity. Creative Child and Adult Quarterly 1987; 12: 237–48.

Sheldon KM. Creativity and goal conflict. Creativity Research Journal 1995; 8: 299–306.

Sternberg RJ (ed.). Handbook of Creativity. Cambridge: Cambridge University Press, 1999.

Thompson M, Blair SEE. Creative arts in occupational therapy: ancient history or contemporary practice? Occupational Therapy International 1998; 5: 49–65.

Trent DR (ed.). Mental Health Promotion. Aldershot: Gower, 1992.

Tudor K. Mental Health Promotion. Paradigms and Practice. London: Routledge, 1996.

United Nations. World Population Prospects: The 2002 Revision and World Urbanization Prospects: The 2001 Revision. Population Division of the Department of Economic and Social Affairs of the United Nations Secretariat, 2002. (Accessed March 2002: http://esa.un.org/unpp/p2k0data.asp)

Vessels G. The creative process: an open-systems conceptualisation. Journal of Creative Behaviour 1982; 16: 185–95.

West MA, Rickards T. Innovation. In: Runco MA, Pritzker SR (eds), Encyclopedia of Creativity (Vol. 2). London: Academic Press, 1999; 45–55.

Wilcock AA. An Occupational Perspective of Health. Thorofare, NJ: Slack, 1998.

Wilcock AA. Occupation for Health. Volume 1. A Journey from Self-health to Prescription. London: British Association of Occupational Therapists, 2001.

World Health Organization. Constitution of the World Health Organization. Geneva: WHO, 1946. (Accessed March 2003: http://whqlibdoc.who.int/hist/official_records/constitution.pdf)

World Health Organization. Ottawa Charter for Health Promotion. First International Conference on Health Promotion, Ottawa, 21 November 1986 (WHO/HPR/HEP95). (Accessed April 2004: www.who.int/hpr/NPH/docs/ottawa_charter_hp.pdf)

World Health Organization. World Health Report 2001. Mental Health: New Understanding, New Hope. Geneva: WHO, 2001a. (Accessed March 2003: www.who.int/whr2001)

World Health Organization. Definition of Mental Well-being. (Factsheet no. 220). Geneva: WHO, 2001b. (Accessed April 2004: www.who.int/mediacentre/factsheets/fs220/en/print.html)

World Health Organization. Depression. (Factsheet). Geneva: WHO, 2002a. (Accessed March 2003: www.who.int/mipfiles/1956/Depression.pdf)

World Health Organization. Facts about Aging. Geneva: WHO, 2002b. (Accessed March 2003: www.who.int/hpr/aging/index.htm)

Zinker J. Creative Process in Gestalt Therapy. New York, NY: Brunner/Mazel, 1977.

CHAPTER 2

A theory of creativity: an innate capacity

THERESE SCHMID

Introduction

Complex layers of centuries of sociocultural behaviour and values have led to the devaluing of creativity in everyday activities and the natural links between creativity and health. The purpose of this chapter is to disentangle and examine those layers, to eliminate some of the present-day complexities associated with the word *creativity* and its meaning, and to highlight creativity as a constructive, viable and contemporary force in daily activities and occupations, which can be consciously utilized to contribute to health and well-being.

Understanding creativity as an innate need is worthy of further study because of its enormous potential. The knowledge to be gained could assist us in sustaining individuals and communities, through being in tune with natural creative biological capacities, sociocultural needs, activity and occupational needs, and the effect of these on health and well-being. This chapter examines early human behaviour and how it has ensured our present day survival as a species. The following discussion provides an opportunity to perceive creativity, and its role in human life, afresh.

Introducing the theory

The theory proposed in this chapter is:

> Humans have both the innate capacity to be creative and the biological need to express it. When creativity is adequately expressed through everyday activities, it has a major impact on health and well-being.

The views expanded upon here, which form a basis of the theory, spring mostly from a range of philosophies and ideas from humanistic, cognitive and educational psychology, neuroscience, neuroanatomy, occupational science, open systems theory, holistic approaches to human health and health promotion, research in creative behaviour, the arts, community cultural approaches to the arts, and art therapy. These will be discussed in relation to recent findings from the new fields of study about the origins of human nature and behaviour: palaeoanthropology, cultural anthropology and evolutionary psychology.

Key concepts will be defined, and the framework for the theory is described. Creativity will then be introduced as a major driving force in the evolution of human nature, linked to health and well-being through the pressure to adapt and survive. Current findings from palaeoanthropology and associated literature reveal that humans evolved significantly 40–50,000 years ago and that there was a shift in human behaviour. The shift in human behaviour is illustrated by describing the shift in anatomical structures, biological and physiological mechanisms, and in the socioculture. Creativity is then described as an outcome of the interchange between these phenomena, the same interchange that resulted in the modern human mind. The manner of that described evolution is a significant basis for this theory, connecting creativity with 'health and well-being'. The health and well-being of humans in the Upper Palaeolithic period will be discussed. It will be shown that, during that period, creativity was integral to everyday activities and occupations. Theories of human nature are discussed in order to establish creativity as an innate need. A discussion about 'what is wrong with everyday activities' in the present time will demonstrate that, in relatively recent years, the demand for and expression of creativity in the everyday activities and occupations of individuals has waned, with significant consequences. The final section will briefly discuss possible ways in which creativity may be restored as an everyday opportunity to improve the quality of life and health; these will be discussed in some detail in Chapter 10.

Key concepts

Several key concepts serve as a backdrop to the ideas in this theory. They are creativity, everyday creativity, innovation, survival, adaptation, culture, health and well-being. These are defined and described as follows.

Creativity

Many definitions of creativity have been offered, including those in Runco and Pritzker's (1999) *Encyclopedia of Creativity*, but these do not fully support the argument of this book. Although supporting the claim of Australian social scientist Colin Peile (1994) that creativity is fundamental to all processes, for the purposes of this chapter, creativity is described and defined, as stated in Chapter 1:

> Creativity is the innate capacity to think and act in original ways, to be inventive, to be imaginative and to find new and original solutions to needs, problems and forms of expression. It can be used in all activities. Its processes and outcomes are meaningful to its user and generate positive feelings.

Creativity is a special kind of thinking process. It requires the ability to conceptualize outcomes from actions, which enables innovative productivity in most fields of endeavour. It is also the basis for various forms of celebration activity. Within this chapter, discussions about creativity are limited to that which is positive or beneficial to users and society. The author acknowledges that there are forms of creativity that are destructive (Peile, 1994).

Everyday creativity

In modern Western society the word *everyday* has often been associated with the mundane or ordinary. Perhaps this is because the dictionary meaning is 'commonplace' (*see* the *Concise Oxford Dictionary*, Pearsall, 1999). In the context of the theory in this chapter, *everyday* has a high-value meaning, which is that all everyday activities can be valuable and meaningful. Creativity can be part of making that so. Because of the mundane view of the word *everyday*, the apparent value of everyday creative activity is diminished. The implication is that the only kind of creative activity worth researching and discussing is the 'special kind', the kind that belongs to 'talented and gifted people'. A challenge to these notions has been expressed by various writers from a number of different fields of research (Ripple, 1989; Cropley, 1990; Richards, 1999), and especially by women such as American artist and art educator, Betty Edwards (1979, 1986), American occupational therapist, Betty Hasselkus (2002), Australian author, Drusilla Modjeska (1999) and English health research writer, Frances Reynolds (2000; *see also* chapters 5 and 6).

Innovation

The *Concise Oxford Dictionary* (Pearsall, 1999) defines *innovation* as 'a creative outcome in which changes are made in something that already existed, as by the introduction of new methods, ideas or products'.

Survival

The *Concise Oxford Dictionary* (Pearsall, 1999) defines *survive* as 'continue to live or exist'. It defines 'survival of the fittest' as, 'the continued existence of organisms best adapted to their environment; natural selection'. Survival is the primary drive of humans and of animals. Survival is dependent upon the capacity to be creative (or adaptive) through occupations and activities. Through their creative capacities, humans developed technology and culture by participating in many activities and occupations which were related to the maintenance and survival of individuals, groups and communities. That maintenance and survival implies health and well-being.

Adaptation

In this chapter, *adaptation* means a part of the human creative process involving the creative use of, or response to, the environment. That is, an individual or group consciously chooses to make a change to suit a new environment (Hagedorn, 1997). Similarly, the *Concise Oxford Dictionary* (Pearsall, 1999) defines *adapt* as 'to make suitable for a new use or purpose'. It defines *adaptation* as 'a change, or the process of change, by which an organism or species becomes better suited to its environment'.

Culture

Culture is defined in the *Concise Oxford Dictionary* (Pearsall, 1999) as 'the customs, institutions and achievements of a particular nation, people or group'.

Health and well-being

In addition to the definitions of health and ill-health described in Chapter 1, further definitions are included below that demonstrate that health is a positive response to well-connected relationships between individuals and their communities, culture and the environment. Spiritual well-being should be included in the definition because it is necessary for health and well-being that people be engaged in a meaningful life (Wilcock, 1998). The definitions of health and well-being incorporate an occupational perspective of health; that is, occupation is the natural biological mechanism for health and well-being (Wilcock, 1998, 2001). In other words, it is through occupations and activities that health and well-being are experienced and affected.

The Australian indigenous notion of health and well-being reveals the importance of culture, the environment, harmony and interconnection. Health and health promotion were defined in the 1989 Australian National Aboriginal Health Strategy as:

> Not just the physical well-being of an individual, but . . . the social, emotional and cultural well-being of the whole community in which each

individual is able to achieve their full potential as a human being thereby bringing about the total well-being of their community. It is a whole-of-life view and includes the cyclical concept of life–death–life. (Commonwealth Department of Health and Aged Care, 2000, p. 83)

and:

The Aboriginal Mental health promotion must incorporate all aspects of well-being; physical, social, cultural, emotional and spiritual . . . Aboriginal essence lies at the heart of cultural well-being. It is shaped and expressed in the web of physical, spiritual, political, environmental, economic and ideological interrelations. Cultural well-being is the outcome of the integrity and harmony of these inter-relations. These inter-relations operate at the individual, family, community and societal levels. (Commonwealth Department of Health and Aged Care, 2000, p. 83)

Perspectives of transpersonal views of global health and ecological issues echo the above notions of health, where there is a deep ecological concern for the whole of nature, including human beings. Health appears to be connected to 'the shift from thinking of the self as a separate, independent entity to recognising its complete interdependence in the totality' (Vaughan, 1985; as cited in do Rozario, 1997, p. 116).

Framework for the theory

The theory proposed in this chapter is that:

Creativity is an innate capacity in humans which, when expressed through everyday activities, has a major impact on health and well-being.

This is both philosophical and practical. *Theory* is defined in the *Concise Oxford Dictionary* (Pearsall, 1999) as 'a system of ideas intended to explain something, especially one based on general principles independent of the thing to be explained'. The theory in this chapter will be supported by an open systems approach because it is built upon the belief that creativity and health are dynamic, interactive and holistic complex phenomena. Diverse branches of enquiry will be used to identify, describe and explain human creative capabilities and behaviour. This will clarify the relationship between creativity and health.

An open systems approach is used to study human behaviour and to identify and explain the characteristics and processes of complex living phenomena (van Bertalanffy, 1968). It recognizes interactions between living phenomena and the environment, and the actualization of potential (van Bertalanffy, 1968; as cited in Kielhofner, 1985). In application to humans, the interactive systems are both internal and external. The complex internal system consists of the biological system, the cognitive mechanisms and the physiological systems supporting emotions. The essential external systems consist of the social environment, including culture, and the physical environment. The internal and external environments or components continually interact, and through processes of feedback, actualize human potential. An important aspect of an open system approach is that it seeks 'to study humans as gestalt wholes recognizing that human behaviour cannot be understood solely by studying underlying components' (Kielhofner, 1985, p. 4). An open systems approach is widely applied in the study of human behaviour and health (Kielhofner, 1985; do Rozario, 1997). This approach is relevant to the study of creativity, in that creativity is perceived as a behavioural phenomenon, and consists of interactions with the external environment (Csikszentmihalyi, 1990, 1995). Arthur Koestler (1976) promoted this approach in his richly documented study of artistic creation.

In addition, this theory builds on Australian occupational scientist Ann Wilcock's occupational theory of human nature, which is based on the idea that humans have an innate biological drive to engage in occupation, which she describes as 'all purposeful human activity' (Wilcock, 1998, p. 22). It is also based, in part, on the notion of American occupational therapist Estelle Breines (1995; see also Chapter 3) of occupational genesis, which describes the evolution of occupations.

Creativity has played a major part in activities and occupations. Creativity has been overlooked in most theories of human nature (as has occupation, according to Wilcock, 1998). In addition, the links between creativity and occupation have suffered the same fate. Creativity has played an unconscious part in many occupations and activities, but it is important that it should play a conscious role because of the benefits to be won.

Further, this theory sits within a framework of scientific and evolution theories of the universe and human nature. Current scientific thought generally supports the view that 'living matter evolved naturally from non-living matter in the form of single celled creatures' (Wilcock, 1998, p. 28) and supports the truth of Darwin's theory that natural selection is the continued existence of organisms best adapted to their environment. That adaptation implies appropriate health for survival. That ability to adapt is probably the origin of creativity.

The following section overviews the early history of *Homo sapiens* and the ability to adapt that has enabled us to survive.

The foundation of creativity: the Upper Palaeolithic period

Cultural anthropological, palaeoanthropolgical, evolutionary biological and archaeological researchers generally agree that human behaviour significantly shifted during the Upper Palaeolithic period, around 40–50,000 years ago (Mellars and Stringer, 1989; Lewin, 1998). For the purposes of this discussion, it is not necessary to enter into the contemporary debate on whether the change commenced abruptly or was the result of an accumulation of changes up to that time. In essence, the theory proposed in this chapter is derived from two premises discussed widely within palaeoanthropological literature (Mellars and Stringer, 1989; Lewin, 1998).

The central premise is that the modern mind of *Homo sapiens* (the primate species to which modern humans belong) evolved during the Upper Palaeolithic period (Lewin, 1998). The term *mind* refers to the information-processing function of the brain (Cosmides et al., 1995). The term '*modern human mind*', within this premise, is taken from an explanation, given by Klein (1992; as cited in Lewin, 1998, p. 116), that the transformation during the Upper Palaeolithic period was 'the last of a long series of biologically based advances in human mental and cognitive capacity'. It is proposed here that the evolutionary causes of this '*modern mind*' and its information-processing functions were the result of the creative human occupations which were necessary for health and survival.

The second premise is that *Homo sapiens* achieved this point in evolution because there was major permanent change in the biological architecture in the brain (Lewin, 1998). The word *brain* is described by neuroscience as the interactions of its physical components, and in psychological terms as 'a system that processes information . . . it takes sensorily derived information from the environment as input, performs complex transformations on that information, and produces either data structures (representations) or behaviour as output' (Cosmides et al., 1995, p. 8). These premises will be expanded in the following section by describing the shift in human behaviour, specifically the shifts in biological, anatomical structures and the shifts in socioculture.

Although there is disagreement on the cause of this change of behaviour, that is, whether the cognitive change was a result of a biological change or a shift in social organization (Davey and Halliday, 1994; Lewin, 1998), it is accepted here that cognitive mechanisms came into place and enabled creativity capacity. The change in human behaviour involved both biology and culture. Both systems affected one another, and therefore issues addressed in this discussion must take both into account.

Shift in human behaviour

The beginning of the Upper Palaeolithic period is commonly cited as the beginning of 'modern human behaviour' (Mellars and Stringer, 1989; Lewin, 1998). Lewin (1998, p. 119) observed that until the Upper Palaeolithic period there was a lack of innovation, but during the Middle to Upper Palaeolithic transition there appeared to be 'a shift'. He suggested that significant behavioural change was reflected in an 'unprecedented variability in artefact assemblages' (Lewin, 1998, p. 119). For example, there was 'an explosion in the creativity of tool production, and an expansion in the use of raw materials, and new traditions followed closely on each other' (Lewin, 1998, p. 119). These views are supported by Lumsden (1999) and Mellars and Stringer (1989). The abrupt change was manifested in found objects, such as fine tools made out of bone, antlers and ivory. Flake technology was replaced by blade technology. According to Lewin (1998), the design of the tools reflected intended purpose and actual capability. Moreover, Lewin (1998) and Mellars and Stringer (1989) suggested that the evidence in tools and artefacts, and subsequent social changes in human behaviour, indicated that more complex and highly structured cognitive systems had developed and that the change was biologically driven rather than being the product of a cultural revolution.

Shift in anatomical structures

Fossil and archaeological evidence has identified anatomical differences between 'archaic' humans and the 'modern' humans of around 40,000 years ago (Mellars and Stringer, 1989; Lewin, 1998). The evidence led scientists (Mellars and Stringer, 1989; Wilcock, 1998) to describe the differences in relation to gait, pelvis, size and flexibility, precision of the hands, and improved manipulative skills. This alone would have given modern man an advantage over archaic man (Neanderthal and other premodern species). Lewin (1998) supported Trinkaus's suggestion that 'archaic humans' adaptive strategy was anchored in strength, while modern humans relied more on skill. Clever use of tools took the place of brute force' (Lewin, 1998, p. 130).

Shift in socioculture

The radical transformation also involved a shift in social organization (Mellars and Stringer, 1989; Lewin, 1998). People were coming together in larger groups. At this time, there was a 'substantially more intense social milieu, manifestation in larger living sites, a greater density in sites and long distance contacts' (Lewin, 1998, p. 131). This describes significant change, which implies that there was an economic shift in culture and subsistence. For example, evidence has revealed that long distance trade and political connections were being formed (Lewin, 1998). This was the time of the first cave paintings; the time when body decoration began, and therefore the first appearance of artistic expression (Mellars and Stringer, 1989; Lewin, 1998). Archaeologists uncovered large numbers of beads and a musical instrument (Lewin, 1998).

Lewin (1998) suggested that the shift in human behaviour (biological and social) was caused by biological change in the brain, enabling the development of language, and that language is the sole cognitive innovation driving the origin of modern humans. It is suggested that language was only one of many cognitive capacities that was unfolding at that time, including imagination and creativity.

Creativity: an outcome of the interchange between biological mechanisms and social interactions – the birth of culture

The function within an open systems model is circular. In other words, the open system increasingly becomes what it does (Kielhofner, 1985, p. 6). For example, the more that muscles are worked, the stronger they become; the more a person engages in problem solving, the better at it they become. Viewing creativity through this perspective, the more that people applied their new creative capacities, the more successful they became at it, so the more they practised it. Creative behaviour became a way of life. People honed their skills through degrees of self-determination and the necessary adaptation to the environment. Culture grew from the constant dynamic use of creative capacities in interaction with the environment, especially the social environment. Culture grew partly from the sharing of knowledge of the creative behaviours and occupations used for survival and partly from the intra-group and inter-group creative arts activities, which were forms of celebration (for example, the cave paintings, the body decorations and the musical instruments). People became increasingly innovative. Creativity and innovation are interdependent. This intense activity pressured the internal human system to respond, to see new possibilities and to implement many changes. This, in turn, promoted health and well-being, which were at the root of all activities.

Emotions, self-esteem, language, celebration

The emotions (the affective states) of *Homo sapiens* in that time must have been powerful. The Biological, cognitive mechanisms had enabled them to solve numerous problems, and this would have released extraordinary feelings of pleasure and excitement. The extraordinary emotions and the realization of the need to exchange details of new ways to support survival would have caused an urgency to find a language. When people discover they can do something for the first time, they like to share the joy and excitement, and often the details of what they have discovered, with others. This release of emotions, and the joy and excitement of discovery, led to the development of various creative arts and celebration activities. These, in turn, fostered people's self-esteem, their identity with others, a sense of health and well-being and, consequently, the flourishing of culture.

Homo sapiens increased in numbers, and other human species died out (Mellars and Stringer, 1989; Lewin, 1998). This increase in population may have resulted 'from greater efficiency at harvesting limited resources' (Lewin, 1998, p. 135). More people could be fed over a longer period. A wider variety of food, and hence of nutrients, might have been available. At this time 'accomplished hunters lived in larger settlements' (Lewin, 1998, p. 120). This implies a shift in social interchange whereby more people were able to discuss hunting techniques, in turn, enabling people to work together to provide food. That meant that there was plenty of food, leaving some people to concentrate on other activities, other occupational forms of survival, for example better shelter and clothing. Neanderthal man did not survive, because as a species, they could not understand what *Homo sapiens* was doing. (It is interesting that the Latin name *Homo sapiens* means 'wise man'.) In other words, the two groups did not have same cognitive, biological and emotional mechanisms in place. *Homo sapiens* grouped together because 'like attracts like'. Language flourished on the newly developed cognitive mechanisms in the brain.

Health and well-being

When viewing these changes from an open systems perspective, the social environment appears to have been a hive of activity and exchange. Health and well-being were linked to survival and safety. Everybody was involved in activities communally, and these activities or occupations catered for innate physiological and biological needs, which in turn maintained homeostasis or balance. Although people were beginning to form larger groups, the hunter–gatherer and nomadic aspects of their lives had health-enhancing qualities. Not only did they have cardiovascular fitness, but their lifestyle also provided them with opportunities, and probably pressure, to think, plan and be creative about their environment and resources, which in turn satisfied their sustainable personal, kin and community welfare. Wilcock (1998, p. 110) explained, 'Survival would have depended on strength created by a cohesive group in combined activity'. The group was valued as an asset that was central to survival. This would have influenced the development of a communal understanding of health rather than an individual view of health.

Creativity played a major role in health through survival, adaptation and safety. People began to actualize creativity, through this 'new' biological capacity, more and more in everyday activities and occupations. People were doing long distance trading, and through that contact, and when they gathered with their close kin and in larger social groups, they shared, discussed and celebrated their latest survival and safety knowledge and inventions. From this actualization in the external environment 'culture' began, and humans developed a 'mindset' concerned with the expression of creativity. Health and well-being were enhanced through creativity, in turn enabling further creative behaviour. It was a period in which the social culture was changing rapidly. Time saved through innovations could be used in new ways. The development of sociocultural expressions of creativity was probably spontaneous; that is, they grew naturally out of feelings of pleasure and excitement at their increasing ease in survival. This mindset enabled an exciting milieu to exist, contributing to the survival of the species through adaptation. Lewin (1998, p. 135) stated 'This exploration of some aspects of behaviour relating to the origin of modern humans . . . reveals the emergence of one key human characteristic; that of ingenuity and innovation particularly in the technological sphere'. This new mind was wired for creativity, thus rendering creativity biologically inherent. This is the description of the modern mind. What they did was good for them. It worked; they were alive! They were alive when they hunted and gathered, they were alive when they built shelters and they were alive when they celebrated. The population of *Homo sapiens* continued to grow at a great rate (Lewin, 1998).

The foundation of creativity: the biological capacity – recent research

Recent research has evidenced that biological and neurological pathways exist for the expression of creativity (Springer and Deutsch, 1981; Myers, 1982; Vessels, 1982; Edwards, 1986; Hoppe and Kyle, 1990; Bogen and

Bogen, 1999). Klein (1992; as cited in Lewin, 1998) implied that these pathways were developing in the Upper Palaeolithic period. The following discussion will examine how this recent research into biological capacities and physiological and psychological characteristics links to the role of creativity in health and well-being. It will also examine the significance of 'needs' and 'wants', and the vital nature of homeostasis. Some are unconscious mental processes; some are not. Their relationship to creativity will be discussed.

As argued in the preceding section, it was during the Upper Palaeolithic period that the biological architecture in the brain had evolved to the degree that significant, substantial, complex pathways enabled fast and effective cognitive and physiological processes (Klein, 1992; as cited in Lewin, 1998). From this it can be assumed that problem-solving acquired a new dimension, and that permanent pathways equipped for creative thinking, associated feelings (affective states) and behaviour, were actualized. The term 'permanent pathways' refers to complex mental mechanisms in the brain, which creativity researchers now generally accept as necessary to enable creative thinking. A wealth of literature exists on creative thinking (Koestler, 1976; Mayer, 1999; Michael, 1999).

Humans now had the capacity and foresight to use creativity. They understood how to improve their problem-solving skills by reflective analysis, by finding ideas, by finding problems and by using imagination. In contemporary creativity research, problem-finding and idea-finding is generally accepted as part of the creative process (Getzels and Csikszentmihalyi, 1976; Jay and Perkins, 1997; Runco and Dow, 1999). The meaning of 'imagination' is taken from Sinnott (1976, p. 108), who described it in this way: 'a new idea arises almost spontaneously in the mind'. He claimed that what made humans truly human was their capacity to cognitively imagine a situation never yet experienced, and picture in their minds something that they had not seen before. These capacities all helped language to develop.

Through the time and processes of evolution, the brain circuitry, involving the two hemispheres and *corpus callosum*, had evolved and was capable of new functions. The corpus callosum is defined as 'the broad band of nervous tissue that connects the two cerebral hemispheres, containing an estimated 300 million fibres' (*Concise Medical Dictionary*, 2002). Since the 1960s, neuroanatomists have been studying the left and right hemispheres, hemispheric exchange and the corpus callosum, pioneered by the work of Nobel Laureate, Roger Sperry, and his associates (Sperry et al., 1969). Research is now demonstrating that the functions of both left and right hemispheres, as well as the corpus callosum, are valuable in the creative process (Myers, 1982; Vessels, 1982; Edwards, 1986; Hoppe and Kyle, 1990; Bogen and Bogen, 1999). Also, neuroscience research has identified bilateral integration, the link between the two hemispheres, as an important feature of health (Hoppe and Kyle, 1990). The phases of the creative act have been documented as information, saturation, incubation, illumination and verification (Springer and Deutsch, 1981; Myers, 1982; Edwards, 1986; Bogen and Bogen, 1999), although recent research implies that the processes may be more chaotic than orderly (Schuldberg, 1999). Bogen and Bogen (1999) attributed the 'incubation' and the 'illumination' stage of the creative act to the right hemisphere. The corpus callosum can transfer high-level function from one hemisphere to another and plays an essential role when, for example, a solution requires the combining of 'dual memory codes, verbal and imaginal' (Bogen and Bogen, 1999, p. 574). Furthermore, the functions of the left hemisphere are described as mechanisms involving external focus, reality testing and language; for example, verbal, syntactical, linear, sequential, analytic, logical symbolic, temporal, digital (Edwards, 1986; Bogen and Bogen, 1999). The right hemisphere functions are described as being non-verbal, perceptual, global, simultaneous, synthetic, intuitive, non-temporal, and spatial (Edwards, 1986). Springer and Deutsch (1981), Myers (1982), Edwards (1986) and Bogen and Bogen (1999) described the creative process by identifying which hemisphere function is connected with the successive stages of the creative process. Table 2.1 gives an outline of the left and right hemisphere functions and the interactions between each hemisphere in each stage of the creative process.

Table 2.1 Brain hemisphere functions and the stages of the creative act

Hemisphere functions	Stages of the creative act
Left hemisphere (external focus and reality testing and language): verbal, syntactical, linear, sequential, analytic, logical symbolic, temporal, digital	First stage: preparation/information and first insight Second stage: saturation (thinking aside, matchmaking, forming analogies) Fifth stage: verification
Right hemisphere: non-verbal, perceptual, global, simultaneous, synthetic, intuitive, non-temporal, spatial	Third stage: incubation Fourth stage: illumination (intuitive, holistic)

Adapted from Springer and Deutsch (1981).

Generally, scientists agree that although the right hemisphere plays a significant role in creativity it does not appear to be well utilized in our society (Bogen and Bogen, 1999). In addition, a wealth of literature from

the fields of cognitive psychology and education has proposed strategies
and approaches to teach people how to be creative (Edwards, 1986;
Bruce, 1989; Mayer, 1989; Cropley, 1999a, to name but four). Some examples are: using analogical models, suppressing the functions of the left
hemisphere by suspending judgement, creating unusual forced relationships, stimulating the incubation or third stage of the creative process,
stimulating the individual's ability to use the right hemisphere by conscious control of electroencephalogram (EEG) patterns, learning
meditation and relaxation techniques, and by developing flexibility in
thinking. This literature reinforces the notions that individuals can develop a certain amount of control over their cerebral involvement within the
creative process and in problem-solving, and also, by implication, contribute to health and well-being through creativity.

The new pathways in the brain (the new flow of creativity) were attributable also to the development, in the Upper Palaeolithic period, of what
we now know as the limbic and reticular formation circuitry (Hoppe and
Kyle, 1990). *Homo sapiens* found themselves able to recognize the value
of their emotional responses to their creative successes (and the sense of
well-being they derived from that) and wanted to repeat and enlarge on
the processes. This practice had the effect of improving and perfecting the
use of the circuitry until it became the natural and common process.
(Neanderthal man was unable to take this step.) Many scholars have
observed that creative behaviour is not just about cognition. It is also about
the accompanying emotions and feelings (Shaughnessy, 1987; Cropley,
1990, 1997, 1999a, 1999b; Csikszentmihalyi, 1996; Bogen and Bogen,
1999; Hirt, 1999; Creek, 2002). Brain researchers acknowledge the mechanisms responsible for the mental and emotional functions of creativity
(Hoppe and Kyle, 1990; Bogen and Bogen, 1999). Emotions have not only
been identified as being associated with the stages of the creative process,
but are also associated with the end result, the product of an activity or
occupation. The sense of achievement upon completing a creative activity
generates a positive sense of self, resulting in a sense of well-being. These
emotions and mental concepts are strongly connected with health and
well-being. A lack of self-esteem, in an individual or group, will diminish
health and well-being. These notions form a strong part of the philosophical basis of many of the health professions, including the occupational
therapy profession (Kielhofner, 1997; Wilcock, 1998, 2001).

Conscious choice: needs and wants

Humans have biological cognitive and associated neuro-affective mechanisms within the brain that can be activated through choice. The

individual consciously utilizes them, for example, when applying creativity in problem-solving. Open systems thinking is humanistic and incorporates the notions that humans have free will and are capable of spontaneous action, reflection and determination.

We have the capacity to ignore our biological needs, or more importantly, to reinterpret them. Wilcock (1998) suggested that many individuals are not able to distinguish their biological needs from wants or preferences, because the complexity of sociocultural evolution makes differentiation difficult and, therefore, alters the apparent significance of biological needs. Because of this, we can explain the purpose of life in abstract ways rather than biological ways, and attribute meaning to our activity, based on sociocultural influences. In this way we can go against the wisdom of natural selection (Wilcock, 1998). In other words, humans are not necessarily conscious of their health and survival needs. They may not be aware that by denying their creative capacities they are denying some of those needs.

Homeostasis

Stedman's Concise Medical Dictionary for the Health Professions (Dirckx, 1997) defines *homeostasis* as, first, 'the state of equilibrium (balance between opposing pressures) in the body with respect to various functions and to the chemical compositions of the fluids and tissues' and, second, as 'the processes through which such bodily equilibrium is maintained'. Homeostasis is a fundamental, unconscious function, for example, to maintain core temperature. To be in balance is essential to human health.

Contemporary literature suggests that the body's need to be in balance is also connected to mental processes, and that need is basically described as the psychological mechanism to seek 'sameness' in what is perceived and received (Wilcock, 1998; Blair and Hume, 2002). Blair and Hume (2002) claimed that when the balance is disturbed, either by external or internal pressures, individuals tend to operate at a higher rate of energy, and, as a consequence, block attention to any psychological or physiological distress. If the pressures continue, individuals can be in danger of either physical or psychological ill-health. Furthermore, Wilcock (1998) described three categories of essential biological needs that are associated with homeostasis and the role they play in the everyday human experience, especially in relation to health and survival: the need to warn and protect; the need to prevent disorder and prompt the use of capacities; and the need to reward the use of capacities. Veenhoven (1984) described those rewards as meaning, pleasure, purpose and satisfaction.

The choice is to be creative or innovative in order to address this need to maintain the necessary balance. It may be that a person cannot, for any number of reasons, be creative in the workplace, but may decide to be creative in another area of life, for example in the garden. This activity may give balance to that individual's life in terms of autonomy, satisfaction, self-esteem, well-being and psychological health. Creativity can be consciously applied by people who are in artistic professions, or by those in employment positions which encourage creativity, such as architecture, teaching, science, business or therapeutic situations. These examples are what Peile (1994) would describe as 'trans-creativity' at work, and what Maslow (1962) and his followers call 'self-actualization', or what Rogers (1970) would describe as 'self-realization'. It is where creativity is being used consciously to determine a process or idea or behaviour in order to produce a new outcome. This enables those people to flourish and maintain their balance. By contrast, many people, too often, consciously choose to not exert their creativity. In this case the biological capacity, creativity, is underused and homeostasis is not achieved, which may result in declining health. Also, if an individual does not consciously exercise the capacity to respond positively and creatively to significant life events then well-being will be diminished and the individual may become physically or psychologically ill (Blair and Hume, 2002).

Theories of human nature: links to creativity

A theory about creativity is a theory about a part of human nature. It would be too much to ask that explanations of human nature be clear and unanimous. It is not like that, and nor is the perception of creativity.

What is human nature? Stevenson answered this question:

> This is surely one of the most important questions of all. For so much else depends on our view of human nature. The meaning and purpose of human life, what we ought to do, and what we can hope to achieve – all these are fundamentally affected by whatever we think is the 'real' or true nature of man. But there are many conflicting views about what human nature really is. (Stevenson, 1974, p. 3)

Many well-known theorists, their associates and followers have written about human nature, and their ideas have had a powerful effect upon the society in which they have produced their work and publications. Stevenson summarized with the following apt words, and although stated in 1974 and updated in 1999 (Stevenson and Haberman, 1999), the notion remains the same:

> The theories of the ancient Greeks, especially of their great philosophers Plato and Aristotle, still influence us today. More recently, Darwin's theory

of evolution and Freud's psycho-analytic speculations have permanently changed our understanding of ourselves. And modern philosophy, psychology, and sociology continue to offer further theories about human nature. Outside the Western intellectual tradition there are the ancient Chinese and Indian concepts of man, among many others. Some of these views are embodied in human societies and institutions and ways of life, as Christianity and Marxism are. If so, they are not just theories, but ways of life, subject to change and to growth and decay. (Stevenson, 1974, p. 7)

Although theorists have discussed creativity, including psychiatrist Sigmund Freud and psychologists Abraham Maslow and Carl Rogers, most theorists imply creativity in everyday activities rather than explicate it. Petrovic's (1991) interpretation of Karl Marx's writing on praxis showed that Marx thought of humans as 'free, universal, creative and self-creative activity through which man creates (makes, produces) and changes (shapes) his historical, human world and himself' (Petrovic, 1991, p. 435). That certainly elevates the notion of human creativity, but it is not obvious how his view has furthered research in explicating creativity in relation to health and well-being.

Various publications give an historical perspective of views of creativity. Examples are the chapter 'A history of research on creativity', by Albert and Runco (1999), and the chapter 'The concept of creativity: prospects and paradigms', by Sternberg and Lubart (1999). Kneller (1965) also offered a critique of the history of views, and Becker (2000) examined cultural–historical origins of the association of creativity and psychopathology. Some publications describe innovations in particular societies (Needham, 1975). However, generally speaking, they do not include descriptions of creativity for everybody in everyday activities and occupations. Instead, the descriptions of creativity are usually of 'exceptional' people and innovative products, or behaviour. There are exceptions. The humanistic psychology theorists have explicated the notion of creativity and its relation to health, although in a limited way, via the practice of self-actualization (Maslow 1962, 1971, 1987; Rogers, 1970; Runco et al., 1991; Sheldon, 1995). The humanists have observed that a creative person is one who is fulfilled, is self-actualized and is functioning freely and fully. Rogers (1970) identified the inner conditions of constructive creativity as openness to experience, having an internal locus of evaluation and the ability to play with elements and concepts. He also identified the external conditions that foster constructive creativity: psychological safety and psychological freedom. Psychological safety includes accepting the individual unconditionally, providing a climate in which external evaluation is absent and understanding empathically. Psychological freedom means permitting the individual complete freedom of symbolic expression. However, as yet, theorists have given little attention to discussing the potential of creativity, in everyday activities and occupations, for health and well-being.

Theorists among arts therapists, occupational therapists and some health professionals (albeit few) and art professionals do discuss the therapeutic benefits of specific arts activities (Kneller, 1965; Rhyne, 1970; Kubie, 1979; Landgarten, 1981; McNiff, 1981; Kielhofner, 1983; Levine and Levine, 1999; Atkinson and Wells, 2000; Creek, 2002). Arts therapies include therapies with art, music, dance and movement, and drama. Although most of this literature only describes the therapeutic benefits of the arts in a mental health or disability setting, these fields of study have contributed significantly to the knowledge base of creativity and its links with health and well-being. This is discussed further by Jennifer Creek in Chapter 4. Professionals in the arts, such as Marsden and Thiele (2000), who are involved in individual or community health, are emerging as contributors to the literature. Other contributions come from VicHealth (2002) and the Cultural Development Network (2004).

Theories of occupation (Breines, 1995; Wilcock, 1998) are closer to the theory of creativity proposed in this book than other theories mentioned in this section. Wilcock's (1998) theoretical book, *An Occupational Perspective of Health*, is a study of human nature. It examines humans as occupational beings and demonstrates a three-way link between survival, health and occupation. Breines (1995; *see also* Chapter 3) describes the genesis of occupations from earliest times to the modern era and provides an understanding of the meaning of activity for human survival. The theory of creativity discussed here builds on these notions. It is through occupation and activities that creativity is expressed. It is only one step further to link creativity to health and well-being.

Since the 1980s, an increasing number of new disciplines of research have emerged, which offer emerging paradigms or models of thinking about human nature. Some examples of these are palaeoanthropology, evolutionary psychology, occupational science, sociobiology, cultural anthropology and evolutionary musicology, to name six. In 1997, do Rozario referred to this emerging movement as 'new science'. These numerous disciplines and subsequent published works have argued for new paradigms of thought (Koestler, 1976; Ferguson, 1980; Tanner, 1981; Gove and Carpenter, 1982; Bohm and Peat, 1987; Lewin, 1987, discussing Laudau et al., 1989; Peile, 1994; Barkow et al., 1995; Goodall, 1996; do Rozario, 1997; Wilcock, 1998; Wallin et al., 1999). These emerging fields of thought have a holistic approach, gathering and synthesizing knowledge from a number of diverse and unexpected fields of study, drawing knowledge – sometimes implicitly, sometimes explicitly – from humanistic psychological and general systems theories.

These new paradigms, especially the transpersonal paradigm (do Rozario, 1997), the creative paradigm (Peile, 1994), evolutionary psychology and occupational science, could be vehicles for the further investigation of creativity for health and well-being.

The transpersonal paradigm adheres to the idea of humans going beyond the individualism of human activity to incorporate the transcendence of the self, not only in identifying the self as an ecosystem existing within a larger system, but also, in doing so, thinking of the self as interdependent in the totality of the ecosystem. It is a paradigm that is naturalistic, inclusive and transcendent (do Rozario, 1997). The thinking within this paradigm relates to health in the sense that if the individual does not experience self in this way then 'we get sick, violent, and nihilistic, or else hopeless and apathetic' (Maslow, 1968; as cited in do Rozario, 1997, p. 116).

Peile's (1994) theory is relevant to the theory outlined in this chapter in the sense that he described in detail how creativity is implicit in life, and he also described the various forms creativity takes when it is explicit. For example, he described the creative paradigm as resting on the notion that creativity is a fundamental aspect of all processes and is implicit. In contrast, he explained that creativity is at an explicit level when people are 'talking about creativity being inhibited, or when talking about one process being more creative than another' (Peile, 1994, p. 160). Furthermore, Peile (1994) viewed all processes as creative; therefore, destructive and repetitive processes are creative as well. Peile (1994) described the implications and consequences of the way in which creativity is becoming decreasingly explicit within our society. However, he did not explicate creativity as being a major influencing factor in health and well-being.

Evolutionary psychology studies the social and cultural adaptations in conjunction with the evolved human mind (Cosmides et al., 1995). This discipline has not yet investigated the meaning of creativity. It does, however, focus on adaptation and, therefore, holds the promise of offering new methods of research to the field of creativity and perhaps to health and well-being.

What seems to be wrong? Modern culture has suppressed creativity

Manifestations of creativity can depend on the culture we live in, and to some extent on individual choices. It is a problem that sociocultural values and knowledge are not always directed in the best interests of the health of the individual or the community and, as too often happens, creativity is neglected.

In the modern Western world, creativity is not viewed as part of everyday activities and occupations. Creativity has, also, not been seen as an innate biological capability that we can consciously activate through choice in order to improve our self-esteem, thus benefiting our health and well-being. Instead, creativity has long been subject to sociocultural obstacles. It is widely believed that creativity belongs to an élite and 'talented' few, that artists are expected to suffer mental anguish and actual manifestations of madness (Becker, 2000), and that in order to be 'successful', a creative person (artist/writer/musician and so forth) must enter the competitive material world. Moreover, much has been written about the historical gender bias towards males and the Western notion of genius, which are seen to have devalued and disempowered female creativity (Greer, 1981; Weisberg, 1993; Modjeska, 1999; Becker, 2000). In addition, the mundane view of the word *everyday* has brought a stigma of unimportance to everyday creative activity. These views and beliefs have been obstacles that, over a long time, have inhibited many people from being creative and from enjoying the benefits to health and well-being that derive from creative activity, especially in everyday activities.

Lewin (1987) claimed that there has been no advance in our biological evolution since the Upper Palaeolithic period. Various theorists claim that the speed of cultural evolution has outpaced our biological evolution (Ferguson, 1980; Barnaby, 1988; Barkow et al., 1995; Wilcock, 1998). This is of concern, for we now have a very different environment and culture than we had not only 50,000 years ago, but even 500 years, or 50 years ago. This rapid evolution begs the question: 'Are we living the life we are most suited to when our physical world has changed so much?'. Building on these notions is the idea raised by Wilcock (1998, p. 115): 'as some basic biological needs of humans are now obscured by millions of years of acquired values, present-day health awareness may not reflect needs that were, and probably still are, fundamental to healthy survival.' This concern raises the additional question: do humans have the capacity to survive the 'modern world' without adequately using our present biological cognitive mechanisms? This book was prompted by recent alarming statistics that revealed that depression will become the leading cause of disability and the second-highest cause of the global burden of disease (WHO, 2002). Do these statistics suggest a trend that we are failing to maintain homeostasis, and is that failure partly because we do not engage our potential for creativity? Such statistics have challenged the author to consider where creativity lies within the minds of health policymakers, arts-in-health policymakers, health professionals, educationalists, the general population, the elderly, those who are at risk of developing a mental illness and those who have a mental illness. The truth of the theory developed in this chapter and the state of the global problem of depression, suggests that keeping in tune with our innate biological needs is an essential part of keeping healthy as a species.

One reason that many people are not creative within everyday activities and occupations is because there is no longer a clear pressure to survive, that is, to continue to exist. When people had the pressure to survive, for example, in the Upper Palaeolithic period, they were forced to use their creative capabilities. Now, it seems, there is little pressure to survive except in the war-torn countries of the world. For most of us the key physical issues to do with survival, such as food, shelter, conveniences and appliances, are satisfied. These are all made for us by the efforts of other creative people. If we want these things, we just have to go and buy them, so the pressure has shifted to maintaining our ability to earn money. The result is that over time, especially since the Industrial Revolution, creativity has diminished in everyday activities and occupations. Do Rozario (1997, p. 6) summed this up in the following way: 'It would seem that the technocratic paradigm led by positivistic science, and the humanistic view of the world where individualism and separatism reign, have joined forces in creating modern cultures, environments and lifestyles of alienation and unchecked consumerism.' This view is also expressed by Warren (2001, 2003).

From 40 to 50,000 years ago until the present, humans have continued to excel in their creative capacities, resulting in millions and millions of inventions and creative works of arts, in all spheres and cultures, which in turn enhanced physical survival. Lewin (1987) described these cultural changes eloquently:

> . . . like an arrow through time, evolution has been considered to be engaged in a constant process of improvement of form and function, clever adaptations constantly being honed to be yet cleverer . . . The worship of progress in the world is in fact a feature peculiar to Western civilisation, born initially of the tremendous material advances that accrued through the engines of the industrial revolution. Change, constant change and advancement – this became the operating ethos. (Lewin, 1987, p. 41)

Furthermore, this ethos has continued unabated without revision. It has not only lost its usefulness in keeping the species alive but may be contributing to ill-health in various ways. For example, it is in direct conflict with the notion of homeostasis, especially the psychological mechanism that seeks 'sameness' in order for people to make sense of the world. This is not advocating that there be no change but rather that there be recognition of the innate biological and psychological mechanism for sameness, which is 'a prerequisite for the existence of a sense of self and is central to giving meaning and of appreciating contrast and differences' (Wilcock, 1998, p. 64). These very mechanisms are essential in the treatment of those who are depressed. Being appropriately creative can restore the balance and can help to restore self-esteem and life satisfaction and consequently health, paralleling the health-normalizing benefits of appropriate nutrition and exercise.

Our current Government sees the health determinants of our society as 'multi-causal'. Disease, disability and, ultimately, death are seen to be the result of the interaction of human biology, lifestyle and environment, including social factors, modified by healthcare interventions (AIHW, 2002). But nowhere in the list of social determinants, defined by the Better Health Commission of Australia (1986) in its document *Looking Forward to Better Health*, does creativity appear.

It is now widely known that the factors that define our social group also directly influence the chances of illness or early death (Morin, 2001). Health is closely related to socioeconomic status and, of course, other factors such as justice, social equity, individual rights, ethical concerns, dietary habits, smoking, physical activity and political and economic priorities. When any of these factors are not in balance, people may suffer low self-esteem. The implications are that people need opportunities. One of those opportunities is to be creative.

It is unfortunate to think that social structures can prevent anyone from having the opportunity to reap the benefits of creativity. It is too unrealistic to place the blame on someone else for the lack of well-being. However, because the layers of sociocultural values and knowledge have minimized creativity in our everyday thinking, it is necessary that governments assist in explicating both the value of creativity in everyday activities, and the links, via self-esteem, to health and well-being. It is necessary that governments enable and resource an education process that explains the value of creativity and promotes its daily use. Then it is up to the individual and the community to understand the principles and devise ways to act on them.

Summary

The theory proposed in this chapter is that humans have both the innate capacity to be creative and the biological need to express it. When creativity is adequately expressed through everyday activities, it has a major impact on health and well-being. The theory is based on two premises: that the modern human mind of *Homo sapiens* evolved during the Upper Palaeolithic period, and that *Homo sapiens* achieved this point in evolution because there was a major permanent change in the biological architecture in the brain. In addition, it was proposed that the cognitive mechanisms that came into place within the Upper Palaeolithic period enabled creative capacity, so that creative behaviour became a way of life and enabled survival. In recent times, particularly since the Industrial Revolution, sociocultural behaviour and values have devalued creativity in everyday activities. The choice as to whether to use the creative capacity has been sidelined by the lack of the practical necessity and survival pressure to use it. It has also been sidelined by the sociocultural values that suggest that it is not important enough to be the subject of conscious effort.

This theory is not very complicated. In fact it is the most natural thing in the world. If you have any doubts about the proof by academic argument, then reflect and ask yourself, 'how could it be otherwise?'

Putting the ideas to work

If proper attention is given to the innate creative capability of all people and their need to express it, the community will see an improvement in the health and well-being of all, and, significantly, a reduction in the incidence of depression. This requires understanding and positive action by politicians, health promoters, professionals in health, economics, arts and education, and by communities and individuals. The methods to achieve this will be primarily through education, but also it is vital that the community establishes and sustains group creativity in order to maintain the stimulation of individuals by interaction. It is essential for governments to create the environment and supply the funding to initiate appropriate programmes. These solutions will be dealt with in more detail in Chapter 10.

References

Albert RS, Runco MR. A history of creativity. In: Sternberg RJ (ed.), Handbook of Creativity. Cambridge: Cambridge University Press, 1999; 16–31.

Atkinson K, Wells C. Creative Therapies: A Psychodynamic Approach Within Occupational Therapy. Cheltenham: Stanley Thornes, 2000.

Australian Institute of Health and Welfare (AIHW). Australia's Health. (AIHW Cat. No. AUS-25). Canberra, ACT: Australian Government Publishing Service, 2002.

Barkow JH, Cosmides L, Tooby J (eds). The Adapted Mind: Evolutionary Psychology and the Generation of Culture. New York, NY: Oxford University Press, 1995.

Barnaby F (ed.). The Gaia Peace Atlas: Survival into the Third Millennium. London: Pan Books, 1988.

Becker G. The association of creativity and psychopathology: its cultural-historical origins. Creativity Research Journal 2000; 13: 145–53.

van Bertalanffy L. General systems theory: a critical review. In: Buckley W (ed.). Modern System Research for the Behavioural Scientist. Chicago, IL: Aldine, 1968; 11–30.

Better Health Commission of Australia. Looking Forward to Better Health. Canberra, ACT: Australian Government Publishing Service, 1986.

Blair SEE, Hume CA. Health, wellness and occupation. In: Creek J (ed.). Occupational Therapy and Mental Health (third edition). London: Churchill Livingstone, 2002; 15–27.

Bogen JE, Bogen GM. Split brains: interhemispheric exchange in creativity. In: Runco MA, Pritzker SR (eds), Encyclopedia of Creativity (Vol. 2). London: Academic Press, 1999; 571–75.

Bohm D, Peat FD. Science, Order and Creativity. Toronto: Bantam, 1987.

Breines EB. Occupational Therapy: Activities from Clay to Computers. Theory and Practice. Philadelphia, PA: FA Davis, 1995.

Bruce R. Creativity and instructional technology: great potential, imperfectly studied. Contemporary Educational Psychology 1989; 14: 257–74.

Commonwealth Department of Health and Aged Care. Promotion, Prevention and Early Intervention for Mental Health – A Monograph (PN2797). Canberra, ACT Australia: Mental Health and Special Programs Branch, 2000.

Concise Medical Dictionary. Oxford: Oxford University Press, 2002. (Reference online.)

Cosmides L, Tooby J, Barkow JH. Introduction. In: Barkow JH, Cosmides L, Tooby J (eds), The Adapted Mind: Evolutionary Psychology and the Generation of Culture. New York, NY: Oxford University Press, 1995; 2–13.

Creek J (ed.). Occupational Therapy and Mental Health (third edition). London: Churchill Livingstone, 2002.

Cropley AJ. Creativity and mental health in everyday health. Creativity Research Journal 1990; 3: 167–79.

Cropley AJ. Fostering creativity in the classroom: general principles. In: Runco MA (ed.), The Creativity Handbook. Cresskill, NJ: Hampton Press, 1997; 83–114.

Cropley AJ. Education. In: Runco MA, Pritzker SR (eds), Encyclopedia of Creativity. London: Academic Press, 1999a; 629–37.

Cropley AJ. Definitions of creativity. In: Runco MA, Pritzker SR (eds), Encyclopedia of Creativity (Vol. 1). London: Academic Press, 1999b; 511–24.

Csikszentmihalyi M. The domain of creativity. In: Runco MA, Albert RS (eds), Theories of Creativity. London: Sage, 1990; 190–214.

Csikszentmihalyi M. Society, culture, and persons: a systems view of creativity. In: Sternberg RJ (ed.), The Nature of Creativity: Contemporary Psychological Perspectives. Cambridge: Cambridge University Press, 1995; 325–39.

Csikszentmihalyi M. Creativity: Flow and the Psychology of Discovery and Invention. New York, NY: HarperCollins, 1996.

Cultural Development Network. (Accessed April 2004: www.community-builders.nsw.gov.au/events/20040205_708.html)

Davey B, Halliday T. Human Biology and Health: An Evolutionary Approach. Philadelphia, PA: Open University Press, 1994.

Dirckx JH. Stedman's Concise Medical Dictionary for the Health Professions (third edition). Philadelphia, PA: Williams & Wilkins, 1997.

Edwards B. Drawing on the Right Side of the Brain: A Course in Enhancing Creativity and Artistic Confidence. New York, NY: St Martin's Press, 1979.

Edwards B. Drawing on the Artist Within. Glasgow: Fontana/Collins, 1986.

Ferguson M. The Aquarian Conspiracy: Personal and Social Transformation in the 1980s. Los Angeles, CA: JP Tarcher, 1980.

Getzels JW, Csikszentmihalyi M. The Creative Vision: A Longitudinal Study of Problem Finding in Art. New York, NY: Wiley, 1976.

Goodall J. Occupations of chimpanzee infants and mothers. In: Zemke R, Clark F (eds), Occupational Science: The Evolving Discipline. Philadelphia: FA Davis, 1996; 31–42.

Gove WR, Carpenter GR (eds). The Fundamental Connection between Nature and Nurture: A Review of the Evidence. Toronto: Lexington Books, 1982.

Greer G. The Obstacle Race. London: Picador, 1981.

Hagedorn R. Foundations for Practice in Occupational Therapy. London: Churchill Livingstone, 1997.

Hasselkus BR. The Meaning of Everyday Occupation. Thorofare, NJ: Slack, 2002.

Hirt ER. Mood. In: Runco MA, Pritzker SR (eds), Encyclopedia of Creativity (Vol. 1). London: Academic Press, 1999; 241–50.

Hoppe KD, Kyle NL. Dual brain, creativity and health. Creativity Research Journal 1990; 3: 150–7.

Jay ES, Perkins DN. Problem finding: the search for mechanism. In: Runco MA (ed.), The Creativity Research Handbook (Vol. 1). Cresskill, NJ: Hampton Press, 1997; 257–93.

Kielhofner G (ed.). Health Through Occupation: The Theory and Practice in Occupational Therapy. Philadephia, PA: FA Davis, 1983.

Kielhofner G. A Model of Human Occupation: Theory and Application. Philadelphia, PA: Williams & Wilkins, 1985.

Kielhofner G. Conceptual Foundations of Occupational Therapy (second edition). Philadephia, PA: FA Davis, 1997.

Kneller GF. The Art and Science of Creativity. New York, NY: Holt, Reinhart & Winston, 1965.

Koestler A. The Act of Creation. London: Hutchinson of London, 1976.

Kubie LS. Neurotic Distortion of the Creative Process. Toronto: McGraw-Hill Ryerson, 1979.

Landgarten HB. Clinical Art Therapy. New York, NY: Brunner/Mazel, 1981.

Levine SK, Levine EG (eds). Foundations of Expressive Arts Therapy: Theoretical and Clinical Perspectives. London: Jessica Kingsley, 1999.

Lewin R. Bones of Contention. New York, NY: Simon & Schuster, 1987.

Lewin R. Origins of the Modern Humans. New York, NY: Scientific Library, HPHLP, 1998.

Lumsden CJ. Evolving creative minds: stories and mechanism. In: Sternberg RJ (ed.), The Handbook of Creativity. Cambridge: Cambridge University Press, 1999; 153–68.

Marsden S, Thiele M (eds). Risking Art. Art for Survival: Outlining the Role of the Arts in Services to Marginalised Young People. Melbourne, Victoria: Jesuit Social Services, 2000.

Maslow AH. Toward a Psychology of Being. Princeton, NJ: Van Nostrand, 1962.

Maslow AH. The Farther Reaches of Human Nature. New York, NY: The Viking Press, 1971.

Maslow AH. Motivation and Personality (third edition). New York, NY: Harper & Row, 1987.

Mayer RE. Cognitive views of creativity: creative teaching for creative learning. Contemporary Educational Psychology 1989; 14: 203–11.

Mayer RE. Problem solving. In: Runco MA, Pritzker SR (eds). Encyclopedia of Creativity (Vol. 2). London: Academic Press, 1999; 437–47.

McNiff S. The Arts and Psychotherapy. Springfield, IL: Charles C Thomas, 1981.

Mellars P, Stringer C (eds). The Human Revolution: Behavioural and Biological Perspective on the Origins of Modern Humans. Edinburgh: Edinburgh University Press, 1989.

Michael WB. Guilford's view. In: Runco MA, Pritzker SR (eds). Encyclopedia of Creativity (Vol. 1). London: Academic Press, 1999; 785–97.

Modjeska D. Stravinski's Lunch. Sydney: Picador Pan Macmillan, 1999.

Morin P. Symptoms, dreaming and society: process-oriented symptom work as a new approach to illness and disease. Journal of Process Oriented Psychology 2001; 8: 25–33.

Myers JT. Hemispheric research: an overview with some implications for problem solving. Journal of Creative Behaviour 1982; 16: 197–211.

Needham J. Science and Civilisation in China (Vol. 1). Cambridge: Cambridge University Press, 1975.

Pearsall J (ed.). Concise Oxford Dictionary (10th edition). Oxford: Oxford University Press, 1999.

Peile C. The Creative Paradigm: Insight, Synthesis and Knowledge Development. Sydney, NSW: Avebury, 1994.

Petrovic G. Praxis. In: Bottomore T (ed.), A Dictionary of Marxist Thought (second edition). Oxford: Blackwell, 1991.

Reynolds F. Managing depression through needlecraft creative activities: a qualitative study. The Arts in Psychotherapy 2000; 27: 107–14.

Rhyne J. The gestalt art experience. In: Fagan J, Shepherd IL (eds), Gestalt Therapy Now. New York, NY: Harper & Row, 1970; 274–284.

Richards R. Everyday creativity. In: Runco MA, Pritzker SR (eds), Encyclopedia of Creativity (Vol.1). London: Academic Press, 1999; 683–689.

Ripple RE. Ordinary creativity. Contemporary Educational Psychology 1989; 14: 189–202.

Rogers CR. Toward a theory of creativity. In: Vernon PE (ed.), Creativity: Selected Readings. Harmondsworth: Penguin, 1970; 137–51.

do Rozario L. Shifting paradigms: the transpersonal dimensions of ecology and occupation. Journal of Occupational Science 1997; 4: 112–18.

Runco MA, Dow G. Problem finding. In: Runco MA, Pritzker SR (eds), Encyclopedia of Creativity (Vol. 2). London: Academic Press, 1999; 433–5.

Runco MA, Ebersole P, Mraz W. Creativity and self-actualisation. Journal of Social Behaviour and Personality 1991; 6: 161–7.

Runco MA, Pritzker SR (eds). Encyclopedia of Creativity (vols 1 and 2). London: Academic Press, 1999.

Schuldberg D. Chaos theory and creativity. In: Runco MA, Pritzker SR (eds), Encyclopedia of Creativity (Vol. 1). London: Academic Press, 1999; 259–72.

Shaughnessy MF. Health through creativity. Creative Child and Adult Quarterly 1987; 12: 237–48.

Sheldon KM. Creativity and goal conflict. Creativity Research Journal 1995; 8: 299–306.

Sinnott EW. The creativeness of life. In: Vernon PE (ed.), Creativity: Selected Readings. Harmondsworth: Penguin, 1976; 107–15.

Sperry RW, Gazzaniga MS, Bogen JE. Interhemispheric disconnection. In: Vinken PJ, Bruyen GW (eds), Handbook of Clinical Neurology (Vol. 4). Amsterdam, North-Holland: Elsevier Science, 1969; 273–90.

Springer SP, Deutsch G. Left Brain, Right Brain. San Francisco, CA: WH Freeman, 1981.

Sternberg RJ, Lubart TI. The concepts of creativity: prospects and paradigms. In: Sternberg RJ (ed.), Handbook of Creativity. Cambridge: Cambridge University Press, 1999; 3–15.

Stevenson L. Seven Theories of Human Nature. Oxford: Clarendon Press, 1974.

Stevenson L, Haberman DL. Ten Theories of Human Nature (third edition). Oxford: Oxford University Press, 1999.

Tanner NM. On Becoming Human. Cambridge: Cambridge University Press, 1981.

Veenhoven R. Conditions of Happiness. Dordrecht: D Reidel, 1984.

Vessels G. The creative process: an open-systems conceptualisation. Journal of Creative Behaviour 1982; 16: 185–95.

VicHealth. Creative Connections: Promoting Mental Health and Wellbeing through Community Arts Participation. Melbourne, Victoria, Australia: Victorian Health Promotion Foundation, 2002.

Wallin NL, Merker B, Brown S (eds). The Origin of Music. London: Bradford, 1999.

Warren W. Reflections on the 'artistic mentality' and personal construct psychology. Paper presented at The Fourteenth International Conference on Personal Construct Psychology, Wollongong, NSW, Australia, 2001.

Warren W. Pragmatism and religion: Dewey's twin influences? In: Fansella F (ed.), International Handbook of Personal Construct Psychology. Chichester: John Wiley & Sons, 2003; 387–94.

Weisberg RW. Creativity: Beyond the Myth of Genius. New York, NY: WH Freeman, 1993.

Wilcock AA. An Occupational Perspective of Health. Thorofare, NJ: Slack, 1998.

Wilcock AA. Occupation for Health. Vol. 1. A Journey from Self-health to Prescription. London: British Association of Occupational Therapists, 2001.

World Health Organization. Depression: fact sheet. Geneva: WHO, 2002. (Accessed 1 May 2003: www.who.int/mipfiles/1956/Depression.pdf)

CHAPTER 3

Occupational genesis: creativity and health

ESTELLE B. BREINES

Introduction

Human beings have been engaged in a long and adaptive evolutionary process. This lengthy process extends from its beginnings in the prehistoric past, through ancient and modern history, towards an unforeseen future. During this process, human beings' lives have changed, as has their world. Influenced by their tangible and social environments, these changes in lifestyle have resulted from the creativity of humankind as they sought to survive as individuals and as a species.

Examining the past, so that we may better understand how people and their world evolved, may help us to improve the ways in which we can affect our further healthy evolution in a world undergoing tremendous and rapid change, a world that offers us great uncertainty, for our very survival is in question. Armed with this information, we may be better able to find creative solutions that will enhance our further health and survival as a species. It is hoped that this knowledge can be used to enhance therapeutic processes.

Toward these ends, this chapter will review various occupations in which human beings have engaged, from earliest pre-history to the modern era. It will consider how human beings applied their skills in a range of tasks 'from clay to computers' (Breines, 1995, p. i) to meet the demands of a persistently changing world.

A distinguishing feature of human beings, in the course of this evolutionary and developmental process, is their ability to manipulate the environment in creative and skilful ways to meet their physical, mental, emotional and interactive needs as connecting and adventurous social beings. This chapter will discuss the role of creativity in enabling humans to engage in a series of evolving occupations, in a process of occupational genesis. It will examine some of the factors that enabled health, well-being and survival throughout this evolutionary process, as well as suggesting

54

factors that are contrary to health, so as to offer some perspective on the relationship between these factors for the future.

Occupational genesis

The earliest proto-human beings are reported, by various accounts, to have emerged from two and a half million (Isaac and McCown, 1976; Haviland, 1994; Panger, 2002) to four million years ago, along the Rift Valley in central Africa, evolving from primates through various stages of hominids, ultimately to become the creatures presently identified as *Homo sapiens.*

Various theories have been proposed about their transition from tree-dwelling ancestors to beings who stood erect and moved about on flat terrain. One explanation of the origins of these early people, perhaps more metaphorical than verifiable, attributes their emergence as erect beings to the nature of the terrain and flora in the region during the time of their origination, and to the influence of this environment on the adaptation of these unique creatures (Washburn, 1960; Washburn and Moore, 1974).

The Rift Valley, where human beings originated, was a savannah of grassy plains along the eastern border of a heavily forested land. This dense tropical forest was an environment in which arboreal primates lived, and it was from these creatures that these curious, erect people, later to be known as 'humans', were descended (Petit, 1999).

Making the transition from life in the trees to life upon the earth, these primates stood erect in the grass, peering above it and beyond to peruse their environment, seeking food while guarding themselves from predators. Over time, the advantages of this erect posture influenced the inheritance of this and associated traits. Relying on their lower limbs for support and locomotion enabled the development of specialized abilities in the upper extremities and permitted them to use their hands in manipulative and creative skills. Their opposable thumb and hand dominance enabled the primates to do many remarkable things with the objects they found in their world (Bower, 2003). Using their upper limbs in purposeful tasks while they moved about on two legs, enabled adaptive survival in their new world, and foretold unique abilities that they would later develop.

The primates' physical features of erectness, bipedalism and opposing thumbs led, in turn, to the development of unique cognitive abilities and communication skills that furthered their competence. Or perhaps these latter traits led to the physical qualities they exhibited, a question that Washburn (1960) posed. In either case, people who could use their hands and minds with skill could devise tools from the natural things that surrounded them. Those who could communicate would transmit their ideas and share their skills, thereby influencing the survival of their kind into the next generation and beyond.

In time, the adoption of oral communication served to inform their offspring and their community. With communication they could share an understanding of the hazards that surrounded them, discuss potential solutions and share ideas that would bring further advantages. They shared knowledge of the location of stands of fruit trees and berry bushes, and the seasons of their ripeness, and of the habits of animals in their migration so they could hunt them communally to feed themselves and their offspring. Language was an advantage for these people. They could plan their hunts and their treks and share new information and ideas. Their community thrived on this knowledge (Ziker, 2003). Language enabled them to provide information from past to current and later generations through a shared oral tradition. Story-telling was incorporated into their lives along with music, song and dance, all of which served as a library of information to be remembered and transmitted.

Taking their memories and ideas with them, the progeny of these early people dispersed widely throughout the world, ultimately covering all the habitable continents. They were exposed to the various climates and terrains. They moved into the mountains and they hugged the shores. Undaunted by cold or heat or hardship, they conquered each season and each change in climate by adapting what they found in nature to meet their needs in the various environments they called home. Their tools were made of every material they found, animal, vegetable and mineral. Their manipulative and cognitive skills served them well in transforming these materials into valuable objects that enhanced their lives and established their culture (Klein and Edgar, 2002).

As they travelled they encountered new terrain, new plants and new animals, learning to live with them and learning to use them to ensure their health, well-being and survival. Each plant and animal was tested for its usefulness in keeping them well. Nothing was wasted. They were the first conservationists. The skins of animals became their clothing, bones became tools and meat served as food. Even the teeth of animals were used as jewellery with which people adorned themselves, thus empowering themselves with the traits of the spirits they respected and feared, as well as providing themselves with trade goods that they could barter for food and other items. As they travelled, their inherent creativity aided them in solving the problems they encountered in the new lands they discovered and inhabited.

Each of the items they needed they created through trial and error, honing their skills and teaching their offspring and their neighbours the methods they devised. As they moved from place to place, diversifying in both language and habits, many different items were devised, some unique and some simply variations. Baskets, for example, are universal in every community in the world. In each community they learned to make them out of different sorts of materials and used them for many purposes. They were made from palm trees in the tropics and from pine needles in the north. Honeysuckle, grapevines, willow branches, reeds and other materials have all been used to make baskets. Whatever grew in their region was manipulated into tools and artefacts for storing and carrying food and other necessities from place to place (De Leon, 1978; Wolfson, 1979).

People ornamented their artefacts, as well as themselves, to reflect the world they saw about them. Different weaving methods were devised, taking advantage of the qualities of the materials at hand, and reflecting the habits of the people. They created designs by interweaving the natural colours and textures of the materials, and when they wanted different colours, they learnt to dye their materials using vegetable matter, insects and other objects from their immediate surroundings. Objects such as beads and feathers were woven into their work. A visit to any museum containing cultural artefacts will illustrate the many different kinds of baskets made throughout the world, demonstrating their regional uniqueness.

In many instances the objects they produced were decorated according to the makers' experiences. Just as the blue of ice influenced the artistry of peoples who lived in the north, red and gold were found in the artefacts of the warmer regions. Symbols of mountains and water, animals, birds and fish – the items of life's sustenance – were inscribed in their work. Artefacts from Asia, Africa, North America, South America and other regions, housed in museum collections, can be observed to differ in characteristics (e.g. American Museum of Natural History and Brooklyn Museum in New York City) (Khouri-Dagher, 1998).

The mud of stream-beds became the clay that was turned into pots of beauty and endurance, as people learnt to master heat (Rossotti, 1993). Clay from different regions has different characteristics. For example terracotta has a red colour whereas other clays are grey. Techniques used to fire pottery differ, creating distinctive pots, such as the beautiful black pottery made by the Santa Maria tribe, which can be found in the Arts and Crafts Museum, New York City (Native Web, 2003).

Controlling fire provided people with food and warmth, and further tools, as they applied it to the world around them (Goudsbloom, 1994). The objects they created were both purposeful and a means of expression, as well as items for sharing and for garnering appreciation from others.

Cold climates required shelters to keep in the heat and keep out the weather; so to live there in comfort, people invented different forms of housing according to the objects and space they found around them. Ice, caves and mammoth bones became their homes (Gladkih et al., 1984). A vivid diorama of such a mammoth bone construction is exhibited in the American Museum of Natural History in New York City, and is described by Jane Auel (1990) in her book, *The Plains of Passage*.

Some peoples used leather from animal skins to create portable housing, turning later to permanent wooden structures as their skills in carpentry developed, and as their tools were invented and refined in a never-ending process of adaptive creativity. John Dewey's Laboratory School, at the University of Chicago, used this evolutionary principle for teaching, drawing on practices of Native American and North American pioneer cultures (Mayhew and Edwards, 1936; Breines, 1995).

Ocean-front environments offered bounty from the sea; so people invented boats and fishing methods and tools to help them feed themselves. Different technologies were demanded for handling trout, salmon or whales. Vessels and tools were created from what grew in the areas they inhabited. In temperate climates, birch bark was sewn into canoes; in the cool rain forests of the American north-west huge cedar trees were hollowed; and in the tropical Pacific islands, pontoons were made from palm and bamboo. Fishing for trout and other river fish required rods made from long and flexible wooden poles, whereas harpoons used for whale hunting needed to be rigid, so the appropriate trees and branches were chosen for these purposes. Nets used for fishing in the oceans and seas were woven from natural products, and differed from region to region according to their availability. Each of these inventive constructions enabled these creative people to travel distances to hunt and fish, taking further advantage of what nature provided. They learned to work together to meet their community's needs.

People needed clothing of different sorts to protect their bodies from the various climates they encountered. They invented these in creative ways, using whatever materials were about them, adapting them for use in each climate. In the deserts, woven cotton gauze provided cover from the sun while allowing breezes through the fabric, whereas wool was used to protect against the cold. People learnt to cure leather and fur, making them into clothing to keep them warm. Silk and cedar, two markedly different materials, one a fragile animal product and one a sturdy plant, formed the basis for the weaving of cloth on either side of the Pacific Ocean. In other regions, wool and cotton, also of animal and plant origins, were spun and woven on inventive looms that were carried from place to place. The garments these people wore reflected their worlds (Lang, 1994).

And so people invented all the means they needed to survive, in all the places that they roamed, influenced by their cultures, developing rules for behaviour from experience, recognizing that their safety and survival depended on the tangible and the intangible; they harvested one and worshipped the other. In time, just as languages differentiated, marked differences emerged in the objects produced by people in different cultures according to the means provided them by their environment, the standards of their families and neighbours, and their understanding of what would keep them safe and well.

Hunters and gatherers who harvested what grew around them ultimately became agriculturalists, farming rice in paddies, and wheat, corn and barley on the plains. They knew what survived best in the world they lived in, and they became experts at growing what they understood. In one location people raised potatoes, in another they grew tomatoes, according to the climate and the season. The climate in Russia, where winters are long and cold, is suitable for growing root vegetables, whereas in Italy, with its Mediterranean climate, tomatoes and zucchini thrive. It is natural that people turned their crops into indigenous food and drink, such as pasta sauce and vodka. Farm produce from different places became a commodity for mutual survival and trade. Recipes emerged which characterized people, some grounded in wheat, some in rice and some in maize.

Nomads became experts in animal husbandry, developing a refined knowledge of the climates in which their animals best thrived. Both flocks and families were moved about to meet those needs. Camels from the Middle East and Africa, sheep from the British Isles and northern Europe, reindeer from the Arctic regions and yaks from northern Asia served the same survival needs, yielding different products and contributing to different cultural identities. Each of the animals raised provided meat and cover to feed and clothe their caretakers, while their caretakers learnt to manipulate the products they provided, turning them into means of furthering life's bounty.

Methods of turning milk into cheese were devised so it would remain a viable food substance, as cheese has a longer 'shelf life' than milk. Many other methods of food preservation were developed as they were needed, for the bounty of one season was countered by the poverty of another. In anticipation of lean times, people learnt to dry meat and fruit, pickle vegetables, make jams and jellies, all to preserve what came in the seasons of plenty, to reserve them for the seasons of want. To assure their bounty, people devised explanations for the seasons, praying for their return in good order, and developing festivals to celebrate these events in conjunction with their tribe.

Methods of spinning and weaving yarn, cotton and hair were developed, all of which retained the same principle, despite the differences in looms and fibres. Yarns were woven under-and-over, the warp and the weft interlocking. Other yarn-craft methods were devised, among them Turkish and Persian knotted rugs, crocheting, macramé and so forth (Short, 1970).

Objects and methods devised in one region found their way to distant lands. Knitting originated in Islamic Egypt sometime between 1200 and 1500 AD. This craft moved to different parts of the world, arriving in Medieval Europe certainly by the thirteenth century (Rutt, 1987; Threads, 1993). What was knitted depended on what materials were available in the regions through which they travelled, while the basic technique remained the same. Two stitches, knit and purl, are all that is needed to create any garment. This process remained the same throughout the centuries, offering functionality as well as comfort in its repetitive action. In the same way, sailors adapted the cords and knots they used when sailing their vessels around the world to create items for their loved ones, or for trade, to while away the long days and nights at sea. Thread, yarn and rope became the basis for fabrics of all sorts, used for all purposes: work, play, leisure and self-care. Clothing, house furnishings, ropes for jumping in play, and yarn used for recreational tasks, were all retained in the human repertoire, satisfying an innate need for creativity.

Newly acquired skills became integrated into the life of each community, satisfying people's health needs and leading to new imaginings and new inventions. With the advantage of controlled fire, people learnt to create metal from rocks, using this knowledge to form tools of ever-greater strength and complexity. Their knowledge of the smelting of copper, bronze and brass was applied to the working of iron, later adapted to the manufacture of steel and more complex metals (Breines, 1995; Cramb, 2003).

Guilds were formed, in which artisans honed their trades and taught their apprentices, who, in turn, became masters of the crafts. Over time, one skill led to another, bringing people from the Stone Age into the Bronze Age, the Iron Age, to an era of industrialization and the modern technologies of electronics, space and science.

New lifestyles emerged to accommodate the changes that came with invention, some of which were healthy and some of which were not. From living in a natural environment, people moved to constructed homes in towns and cities, organizing their labour and their leisure into different time frames, specialized according to education, talent and interest. Ultimately, people came to live in great cities, in tall but vulnerable buildings, creating smog and an unhealthy environment along with their brilliant inventions, risking the health of the populace, yet paradoxically increasing longevity. They moved towards a world in which people who are spread far and wide across the earth, using a diversity of languages, can be in touch with one another within moments through the technologies of radio, television and the World Wide Web. Villages of the past became the global village of the future.

So the same forces and traits that were there at the beginning moved forward in time to meet the needs of people of the modern era, influencing human behaviour and testing their benefit to society for all, albeit in a vastly contracted timeframe. Nor was each invention good for the community. Some societies grew and fell, their success or failure due to a variety of events.

The diseases to which people were subject, shifted and changed. Some of the changes were due to evolutionary mutations and other natural events. Some were due to human efforts with regard to occupation, drugs, immunization, sanitation and transportation. Some were due to the activities in which people engaged. Most were due to the combination of these (La Dou, 1994).

Whilst many activities gradually changed over time, many of them remained the same, although often not for the same survival purposes for which they were originally developed. In many instances, ancient activities, originally designed for survival in one community, became leisure activities in another. For example, the fishing rod, which facilitated survival in one generation, later became a source of leisure and relaxation. These activities provided satisfaction and competence to the masters of these skills, regardless of their origins and purposes (Breines, 1981, 1995). The ancient activities of pottery, leatherwork and yarn crafts remained meaningful when incorporated into culturally relevant activities; so did the later activities, such as carpentry, metal craft and printing, and the more recent ones of website construction and videography (Breines, in press). Each activity fulfils a need that humans have for creative engagement. Choice of activity is dependent on personal interests, desires and talents, reinforced by social commentary and influence. Whether of ancient or modern origin, these activities have filled people's lives and provided personal satisfaction and feedback from self and others.

This process of cultural development has been described as a genesis of occupations, recognizing the unending process of evolution and development in which human beings are perpetually engaged. Occupational genesis is dependent on a mixture of human abilities, of both mental and physical construction, incorporated with the contributions of the environment in which people live, including their tools and space, and a social network whereby communication allows the sharing of knowledge from person to person and from the past to the future. All of these elements together, when combined with the filtering of time and experience, assured the healthy development of the community from generation to generation (Breines, 1981, 1986, 1990, 1995, in press).

Creativity and creative activities

The process of occupational genesis is built on a uniquely human ability: creativity. As we have seen, human beings have a long history of applying their creative abilities to their personal and social survival in unceasingly new and interesting ways. They are the only creatures on earth endowed with this ability. While other beings are able to use tools in limited ways, and other primates (and a few other beings such as dolphins) exhibit certain levels of creative performance, human beings alone have honed this skill to the remarkable levels that enable mastery and foster creative and meaningful problem-solving. It is through this process that civilization in all its forms has evolved.

Many features contribute to creativity. A growing literature of creativity spans a wide variety of topics, which Runco and Pritzker (1999) have compiled into a comprehensive encyclopedia. The largest portion of that literature is devoted to the feature of cognition and its influence on creativity, ignoring the influence of body on this process with one exception, the brain, since it is the role of the brain, as the physicality of the mind, that interests researchers. Scientists who are concerned with creativity have largely ignored the role of the body as performer and the unity of mind and body in task performance. This literature is largely grounded in cognitive psychology, within a Cartesian perspective of the world. The study of creativity seems grounded in a reductionist approach, an odd configuration given the topic.

Also, the literature of creativity exhibits a degree of élitism. The experiences and actions of especially creative people are examined to unlock the mystery of human creativity. Gruber, for example, committed his research to examining the life works of such geniuses as Darwin and Piaget (Gruber, 1981; Gruber and Voneche, 1986). The study of the creativity of ordinary people is limited, deferred to finding out about the creativity of the gifted (McCrae, 1999). The nature of ordinary creativity, those actions engaged in by all people in their usual tasks of living, is largely of secondary interest. The requisite integration of mind and body in creative performance in work, play, leisure and self-care receives limited attention within this literature. Yet, it is of abiding interest to occupational therapists and others who recognize its importance in ordinary human events, and who advance its use as a therapeutic tool. Consequently, examining creativity from the perspective of the ordinary tasks of living, in which all people engage, may be useful in expanding knowledge and skills.

An important and universal relational paradigm is inherent in understanding creativity from this perspective. Creativity is built on a dialectic that is composed of two interrelated phenomena of performance that I have described elsewhere as the automatic and the deliberate (Breines, 1986). An individual's skill in performance emerges from the interaction of these two phenomena, one of which is grounded in the past, and one of which reaches into the future, with implications for both the evolution and creative development of the species.

All creatures are endowed with certain automatic abilities. Some of these automatic abilities are evident at birth as inherited reflexes or traits. Beyond those traits evident at birth, some automated traits are developed in the course of time according to programmed and inherited schedules. Development proceeds according to certain sequenced events. An infant turns its head to its mother's breast to prepare to suck and swallow, thus contributing to its own survival. This reaction to a touch on the cheek is spontaneous and universal among well infants, illustrating the presence of this inborn trait. A series of developmental reflexes follows, and serves as the basis for behaviours that are acquired soon afterwards. We sit before we stand; we stand before we walk; we walk before we run. Each new skill comes in order, although the timing of each new acquisition may vary from person to person. It is not until we have developed past these infantile responses, common to all, that we begin to engage in deliberate, planned behaviours that establish human uniqueness and the creative process (Breines, 1995).

Each of these inherited traits stems from our ancestors, and contributed to their survival, just as it contributes to our own. Each of these inherited traits serves as the foundation for new creative acts in which all humans engage.

We spend our lifetimes acquiring new, often individual, skills that we, ultimately, can perform with some level of automaticity. These are not inherited traits, but rather they are learned performances. However, once learnt, they serve the same functional purpose as those automated traits with which nature has endowed us. Once acquired, they can serve as grounding for creativity and new learning.

For example, consider the activities of driving an automobile or typing. Think how it feels to drive a new vehicle as compared with driving one with which one is very familiar. Driving the new car needs very careful attention. The gearshift stick may be in a different location and have a different feel; the mirrors can be located higher or lower than one is accustomed to; the pedals are in different places and respond to different forces; and the width and length of the car may be different. All of these changes from the familiar require careful focusing at the outset in order to drive safely and they are apt to generate anxiety in the driver. On the other hand, the old car feels comfortable and its components can be largely disregarded. Destination has become the chief focus, as have the plans for engagement at the new location. The familiar can be ignored, and indeed must be, if further skill is to be developed.

A similar phenomenon exists in typing. When we begin to learn to type, all we can think of is the fingering and the location of the keys. However, in time, as we learn to type with speed and efficiency, automaticity is exhibited. Once that automaticity is achieved, the skill can be used toward a more expanded goal, such as writing a report. We are adaptively gifted with the ability to ignore, so that we may learn to function on higher and higher levels of performance, bringing creativity forth. Essentially, this is the foundation of occupational therapists' belief in goal-directed activity as a therapeutic tool. The acquisition of mastery enables creativity. Mastery, on one level, leads to the establishment of goals for achievement on ever-increasing levels of performance. For example, learning to play chess requires that we first know which way each of the pieces move before the game can begin and the tournament won. Preparing a meal depends on our ability to peel, stir, lift and pour before the guests can be invited and the celebration begun.

Examples of human occupation which rely on automatic performance are endless. In fact, they are universal. Every activity in which we engage throughout our life contains aspects of performance that are automatic. With a foundation of reliable automatic performances upon which we can rely we are able to concentrate deliberately and creatively on the solving of problems and the acquisition of new knowledge and new skill. In the alternative, this diversion through creativity strengthens reliable automatic performances on subordinate levels. Invention, the essential result of creativity, may only occur when we have mastery of the necessary underlying skills upon which we can rely.

This integrated motor and cognitive capacity of developing automaticity is fundamental to performance, but it is not the only perspective that must be taken to understand creativity. Creativity is also built on feelings of self-identity and self-confidence that emerge from personal and social experiences of success. Creativity is enabled by the physical and mental abilities that humans bring to problem-solving, and is reinforced by the confidence, or feelings of efficacy, acquired as a result (White, 1959; Fidler, 1981).

Creativity also requires the ability to engage in risk-taking behaviours, in anticipation that risk will foster future success. Without the anticipation of success, there would be no effort. As a matter of fact, stagnancy in taking chances is a sign of ill-health. Healthy humans are continually seeking the appropriate challenge in their efforts to achieve, and their success in these efforts contributes to their personal health and the health of their community. Survival is not a solitary effort; it is a goal of a social group and the result of collaborative effort. Everyone must contribute to the benefit of all, or the group will not survive. We tend to have lost sight of this realization in many instances, as our dependency networks move further and further apart. The extended families and co-workers of the past, who lived close by one another, are now less dependent on one another than before. Ease of travel has placed us distant from one another in many ways (Sullo, 2002).

There must be an underlying drive for people to want to engage in new and stimulating experiences. John Dewey (1929), the great American pragmatist, philosopher and educator, described this driving force as human beings' quest for certainty. He attributed humans' adventurous nature to a quest to understand through action. Furthermore, he indicated that we engage in this process of learning through doing, in an attempt to contribute to society as well as ourselves. Dewey (1916) saw the individual as contributing to society, and saw society's role as contributing to the individual. Certainly, he viewed their participation as being of mutual benefit.

Trying out new ideas is a feature of human behaviour, and underlies the creative drive. These efforts are made in the hope of serving both self and society. Repeating of efforts must be encouraged by at least intermittent experiences of success, hence the appropriate challenge. Creativity is a feature of individual effort, reinforced by social respect and advantage. In addition, creativity can be attributed to group efforts, as ideas are shared when people communicate with one another.

Humans have been endowed with a creative force that they have used over the millennia to solve increasingly more complex and specialized problems. These solutions can be seen in the various forms of expression that have evolved in different cultures. In fact, the people of each culture have developed traditional forms of expression that characterize them. For example, the people of some cultures cover their heads to show respect; others uncover their heads for the same purpose. Food preferences, clothing choices, dances and songs all reflect culture, and vary uniquely among different peoples. The traditional meanings of cultural activities are found within all social groups that unify around these activities. Creativity is visible in each of these activities. It is important to recognize that culture stems from group decision-making. Style and custom derive from adherence to cultural forms. Many of these cultural forms have found their way into occupations in which people engage for work, play, leisure and self-care. Activities such as yarn crafts tend to appeal to women; activities such as football tend to appeal to men. Colouring pictures appeals to children, whereas reading romance novels is an adult activity, and so forth.

While activities, because of their cultural relevance, hold meaning for some, it is also true that where people find that an activity has no cultural relevance, for them it may be meaningless. Careful attention to the relevance of activity for individuals is required, if it is to be used to enhance health and performance. Creativity grows within such an environment, nurtures further growth, and contributes to well-being.

Health and well-being

Health is a term that eludes clear and consistent interpretation. Some consider health to be the absence of physical or mental disease (Hassel and

Hafner, 2002). Others view the term 'health' as more comprehensive and broadly understood (Byrd Program for Integrative Medicine, 2003). They interpret health as including the notion of well-being, and those positive feelings people have about their own well-being, as they engage in life's experiences. Here, 'ill-health' can be defined according to the negative emotional feelings that degrade people's sense of well-being and engagement in life's activities. Still others consider 'health' to be a term relevant to social groups and societies (Kansas Health Institute, 1998). Healthy and unhealthy societies are clearly distinguishable from one another.

In different cultures, depending on the belief systems held, responsibility for the preservation of health is attributed to different sources. Some view health to be the realm of specialized practitioners who are formally trained to treat people experiencing illness. Their practice is limited to certain specified parameters, such as medicine, nursing, occupational or physical therapy and the like, and is sanctioned by society in terms of education and licensure.

Others, in many places in the world, feel that those who have gained their knowledge through personal experience can treat health, for example, in midwifery. In such cases, experience, reputation and trust influence the roles and acceptance of practitioners, rather than official recognition. Such reliance on reputation, built on word of mouth, is more likely to be encountered in third world countries or regions of the world where formalized medicine is not readily available.

Auel's (1990) well-researched and respected series of novels, collectively entitled *Earth's Children*, projects how earliest peoples lived, the information largely built from archaeological research and knowledge of indigenous peoples. Auel described how Ayla, the protagonist, becomes a health-giver by gaining experience from guidance and through trial and error, testing herbs for their effectiveness and gaining recognition among her companions for her knowledge. Other societies grant the role of healthcare to spiritual practitioners. Clergy or shaman, they seek higher authority in pursuing health for those who look to their guidance. Still others feel that individuals have the responsibility and capacity to maintain their own health by engaging in life activities that nurture health and avoiding activities that are detrimental to it.

Regardless of its explicit definition, or the nature of its practitioners, health is a topic of universal concern and a state that people seek throughout their lives, and have sought over the course of history.

Now we will consider meanings of health consistent with the premises put forth earlier in this chapter. In essence, we will examine how, in the evolution of human beings, our natural creativity in developing life's tasks and occupational choices serves as a foundation for achieving and maintaining health.

Certain aspects of health are inherited. For example, as with all living things, self-protective mechanisms, such as bipedalism, opposition and oral communication, which contribute to human health and survival, have evolved by natural selection and are understood to be healthful adaptations. Natural selection, described in the nineteenth century by Charles Darwin (1859), is a mechanism of evolution by which traits that are beneficial to the survival of a species are inherited. While Darwin's work focused on the adaptations of animals of various phyla, including birds and reptiles, his ideas can be applied to understanding the influence of natural selection on the health of human beings. For example, some protective mechanisms are found in the natural immunities that we carry. We acquired these immunities as a consequence of mutations that occurred in earlier generations, and they became inherited traits. If our parents and grandparents inherited adaptive traits from their ancestors, and if they serve as assets to longevity, our own ancestors survived as a result of them. Consequently, we, too, can expect to inherit them, exhibit them, and benefit from that inheritance. Those people who are well-adapted are apt to survive to an age where they reproduce their traits, assuring that their descendants will inherit them, thus positively influencing the population over the course of time.

Survival of the individual or the species is dependent on the inheritance of healthful traits. In fact, research has demonstrated that one of the best predictors for longevity is the age of one's ancestors (Mitchell et al., 2001). On the other hand, maladaptive traits have no advantage in survival. The health of those exhibiting such traits is at risk. In a natural world, such as that in which our ancient ancestors lived, the traits that were inherited, along with the fortuitous nature of their experiences, determined who would live and who would die.

Essentially, those who are well adapted to the environment are likely to live longer than those who are not well-adapted, and the latter are less likely to live to procreate. Consequently, the traits of those who are maladapted will be lost to the gene pool, which may not be an advantage to the individual, but is a great advantage to the species as a whole (Dawkins, 1996).

As we have seen, some inherited traits are universally beneficial. Others are regionally beneficial and they were adapted to meet the needs of life within a particular region. For example, differences in skin and eye colour developed as an aid to self-protection. The more melanin in the skin, such as found in peoples who originated in the sunny regions closer to the equator, the more the skin is protected. On the other hand, people who live in a cloudy climate, or where the sun is low in the sky for months on end, benefit from less melanin in the skin as this trait is apt to permit maximum exposure to the sun and increased vitamin D metabolism.

In some instances, a trait that serves as an advantage in one environment may be disadvantageous in another. One such example is sickle cell anaemia, a serious and painful disease found in people of African origin. Yet, carriers of sickle cell are protected from malaria, an important advantage in a tropical climate where mosquitoes (which carry the disease) are prevalent.

In addition to those direct determinants of health such as immunity or other specialized traits, health can be attributed to other influences. Human beings have the advantage of being able to contribute to their own health through their own efforts. Not only have they been able to rely on natural selection to aid in their inherited survival, they are also gifted with the ability to solve problems creatively to contribute to their adaptive health and survival.

Humans beings created new occupations that impacted on health. For example, learning to harvest food from the wild led to raising crops, bringing with it the greater assurance of sufficient nutrients to build strong bodies. As each new skill was acquired, people were better able to meet their own needs as well as those of their social group.

Many of the actions in which we engage are healthful, just as some are not. Some of these are activities over which we have control. Eating healthy diets, a positive action, and smoking, a negative action, are two such examples of behavioural choices about occupations. The health outcomes of some other voluntary actions may be determined by inherited traits. People in different regions of the world developed specialized adaptations to their food sources. Modern south-west Native Americans, whose ancestral diet was primarily maize, now have a greater incidence of diabetes. This is attributed to their exposure to a diet of the modern culture, which is largely composed of wheat and fat, for which they are ill-equipped by heritage. Asians are reputed to have a higher incidence of lactose intolerance than people whose ancestors raised dairy cattle. Those who maintain a diet that is in keeping with their inherited dietary requirements are apt to retain health, but choices are often difficult when new environments provide resources that are less compatible with inherited needs.

While the inheritance of creativity is often a valuable tool for health, some creative efforts have proved to be unhealthy. Many sedentary occupations, aided by labour-saving devices that are characteristic of the modern world, are not healthy. Obesity in children and adults is a new epidemic. Instead of reducing the labour in occupations, people would be better served by engaging in the active exercise demanded by the labour of early occupations (Laudry, 2002).

Certain physiological conditions are observed to be altered as a consequence of activity. For example, stability of blood pressure is associated with activity, and is more likely to be retained at a healthy level when we are engaged in satisfying activity, just as dissatisfying or stressful activity is associated with elevated blood pressure levels, that contribute to ill-health (New York Reuters Health, 2002; University of Glasgow, 2002). Here again, people can influence their health through their occupational choices. Yet, for some individuals choices may be limited for a variety of reasons, such as cost and availability, culture or interest. People demonstrate satisfaction when they are successful at occupations in which they engage (White, 1959). This satisfaction tends to engender feelings of well-being and the maintenance of health. This belief is at the core of a commitment to therapeutic activity as a means of promoting health.

The ability of human beings to communicate has its role in health and survival for both the individual and the group. When people are able to share ideas and memories, they are able to inform one another about known hazards to health. They devise methods to avoid those hazards, and learn to share other ideas to serve their survival. For example, modern people seem to be coming to recognize the hazards to health of a sedentary life, as more and more people join gyms and engage in sports as weekend pursuits.

Along with creativity, the integration of mind and body in manipulative skills has helped us to move our thinking forward and encourage survival. Certainly, 'active occupation', the term adopted by Dewey (1916) for the activities of life in which people engage, remains of great interest to health practitioners. Time after time, activities that emerged to enable survival have re-emerged, in a different form, to contribute to health. Today, it is common, in many places in the modern industrial world, to see clubs and classes in community centres and vacation sites devoted to traditional and modern activities, meeting the demands of people who find them nurturing. For example, yarn crafts, gardening, woodworking and dancing are of great interest. Each of these activities attracts the attention of the public for the satisfying effects they have, and the feelings of well-being they engender (Reed, 2003). Exactly what contributes to these feelings of well-being has yet to be fully understood.

Perhaps our ancient tendency to function in groups has engendered these feelings. Perhaps the use of hands and mind in collaborative efforts is satisfying. Safety and satisfaction may go hand in hand. One wonders if population health is reinforced by the human desire to work together in mutually satisfying tasks. It may be critical to better understand the importance of groups for their impact on our health.

It is commonly recognized that families provide support to one another, but not everyone has the support a family provides. In our modern world, members of extended families are often great distances apart. Even members of households spend little time together in mutual endeavours, with mum and dad at work and children at school or after-school activities. Perhaps we need to encourage the development of groups with common interests, as alternative social networks, to contribute to a healthy existence.

We currently live in a world undergoing great change, and can have little perspective on what events in our lives are beneficial to our health, because we do not know the long-term implications of the changes we are experiencing. The early years of our evolution led to the natural selection of those who could survive. That took aeons to develop. Now we are not permitted the same extended periods of time to experience what is beneficial to enduring health. On the contrary, people who could not survive through their own efforts are now living long lives because of the efforts of modern medicine and sanitation. However, in my view those lives must also be meaningful or they will not be healthy under any of the standards of health we choose to apply.

Clearly, we recognize that active occupation affects health and survival. What we are less sure of is how that relationship comes to pass. We would be well served to begin examining these questions if we are to continue to survive, and if we are to have the skills needed to bring to the therapeutic process.

Solutions

We have inherited a complex of traits that have been enabled by human creativity. These traits have survived millennia in which we have encountered untold numbers of problems, and solved them, leading us to enhanced health and longevity. However, ours is an unending process of solution seeking. Our inherited problem-solving abilities need to be focused on the questions that face us today, so that we can retain the health we inherited.

A number of health issues that come to mind include: the impact on health of nuclear fuel and weapons; environmental contamination; the impact of drugs on disease mutation; and the potential hazards of genetic manipulation. Yet, these are the problems over which people feel they have little control as individuals, and which create anxiety. Identifying methods of empowerment may be the solution.

Intuitively, it seems that creative active occupation is effective as a means of achieving and maintaining health. That must be the case since so many people seek active creative occupation as a nurturing and satisfying experience. Remember, engagement in creative activity that incorporates mind and body has led to human survival over vast millennia. A steady dose of experiences in which we feel control and satisfaction may be what is needed to provide us with the internal fortitude to address problems that escape our direct solution. Engaging in satisfying activity as individuals and as groups may provide the foundational automaticity that enables creative problem-solving toward a healthy society.

Human occupation in creative activity has enabled health in the past. It is now time to evaluate how to use this human tool to further health, both for the individual and society, so that we may continue to survive and grow as a species.

These seem to be formidable questions, but in fact may be no greater than the questions that our ancestors had to face in each of their generations. Human beings have proved themselves to be intelligent creative beings, capable of finding solutions to problems of all sorts in the past. Now we must prove it for the future. Our species' well-being and survival depends on it.

References

Auel JM. The Plains of Passage. New York, NY: Bantam Books, 1990.

Bower B. The stone masters. Science News 2003; 163: 234–6.

Breines EB. Perception: Its Development and Recapitulation. Lebanon, NJ: Geri-Rehab, 1981.

Breines EB. Origins and Adaptations: A Philosophy of Practise. Lebanon, NJ: Geri-Rehab, 1986.

Breines EB. Genesis of occupation: a philosophical model for therapy and theory. Australian Occupational Therapy Journal 1990; 37: 45–9.

Breines EB. Occupational Therapy Activities from Clay to Computers: Theory and Practise. Philadelphia, PA: FA Davis, 1995.

Breines EB. Occupational Therapy Activities for Practice and Learning. London: Whurr Publishers, in press.

Byrd Program for Integrative Medicine, 2003. (Accessed 18 September 2003: www.hsc.uvu.edu/som/pim/principles.htm).

Cramb AW. Department of Materials Science and Engineering, Carnegie Mellon University, 2003. (Accessed 18 September 2003: http://neon.mems.cmu.educ/cramb/processing/history.html)

Darwin CR. The Origin of Species by Means of Natural Selection. New York, NY: MacMillan-Collier Books, 1859.

Dawkins R. The Blind Watchmaker: Why the Evidence of Evolution Reveals a Universe Without Design. London: Norton, 1996.

De Leon S. The Basketry Book. New York, NY: Holt, Rinehart & Winston, 1978.

Dewey J. Democracy and Education: An Introduction to the Philosophy of Education. Toronto: Collier-Macmillan, 1916.

Dewey J. The Quest for Certainty: A Study of the Relation of Knowledge and Action. New York, NY: Minton Bauch, 1929.

Fidler G. From crafts to competence. American Journal of Occupational Therapy 1981; 38: 567–73.

Gladkih MI, Kornietz EL, Soffer O. Mammoth bone dwellings. Scientific American 1984; 251: 164–72.

Goudsbloom J. Fire and Civilization. London: Penguin, 1994.

Gruber H. Darwin on Man: A Psychological Study of Scientific Creativity (second edition). Chicago, IL: University of Chicago Press, 1981.

Gruber HE, Voneche JJ. The Essential Piaget. New York, NY: Basic Books, 1986.

Hassel C, Hafner C. What can we learn about our health from ancient perspectives? University of Minnesota Extension Service News and Information, 2002. (Accessed 18 September 2003: www.extension.umn.edu/extension-news/2002/LearnAboutOUrHealth.html)

Haviland WA. Human Evolution and Prehistory. Ft Worth, TX: Harcourt Brace College Publishers, 1994.

Isaac GL, McCown ER. Human Origins: Louis Leakey and the East African Evidence. Menlo Park, CA: Benjamin, 1976.

Kansas Health Institute. Healthy Societies: An Overview, 1998. (Accessed 18 September 2003: www.founders.net//fn/papers.nsf)

Khouri-Dagher N. Botswana: The Zebra on Wheels. UNESCO Sources. 1998; 105: 7–9.

Klein RG, Edgar B. The Dawn of Human Culture. New York, NY: John Wiley & Sons, 2002.

La Dou J. Occupational Health and Safety. Itasca, IL: National Safety Council, 1994.

Lang SS. Clothing styles across cultures. Human Ecology: An Interdisciplinary Journal 1994; 22: 5.

Laudry G. The Hottest New Exercise? 2002. (Accessed 19 September 2003: www.practicalweightloss.com/nutritio/articles/the-hottest-new-exercise.shtml)

Mayhew KC, Edwards AC. The Dewey School: The Lab School of the University of Chicago 1896–1903. New York, NY: Appleton–Century, 1936.

McCrae RR. Consistency of creativity across the life span. In: Runco MA, Pritzker SR (eds), Encyclopedia of Creativity. San Diego, CA: Academic Press, 1999, 361–6.

Mitchell BD, Hsueh WC, King TM, Pallin TI, Sorkin I, Agaruala R et al. Heritability of life span in the Old Order Amish. American Journal of Medical Genetics 2001; 102: 346–52.

Native Web. Caveman to chemist projects: fire. 2003. (Accessed 12 November 2003: http://nativeweb.org)

New York Reuters Health. Boring passive work may hasten death. Discussed on Healthline 24 May 2002. (Accessed 6 December 2003: www.drpressman.com/News/news05-02.htm)

Panger M. First primate archaeological dig uncovers new tool development links. Office of Legislative and Public Affairs NSF Press Release, 2002. (Accessed 12 November 2003: www.nsf.gov/od/lpa/news/02/pr0242.htm)

Petit CW. US News and World Report 1999; 126: 17.

Reed D. A perfect circle. Granny crafts help ease the stresses of modern life, 2003. (Accessed 19 September 2003: http://modeweekly.com/2003/03.02.13/03.02.13_a_perfect_circle.htm)

Rossotti H. Fire. Oxford: Oxford University Press, 1993.

Runco MA, Pritzker SR (eds). Encyclopedia of Creativity. San Diego, CA: Academic Press, 1999.

Rutt R. A History of Hand Knitting. Loveland, CO: Interweave Press, 1987.

Short E. Introducing Macramé. Greenwich, CT: Fawcett, 1970.

Sullo E. Long distance families and keeping in touch, 2002. (Accessed 18 September 2003: http://md.essortment.com/longdistances)

Threads. Knitting Around the World, from Threads. Newtown, CT: The Taunton Press, 1993.

University of Glasgow Newsletter. New focus on health and wellbeing. Issue 236, March 2002. (Accessed 6 December 2003: www.gla.ac.uk:443/newsdesk/newsletter/236/html/news16.html)

Washburn SL. Tools and human evolution. Scientific American 1960; 203: 3–15.

Washburn SL, Moore R. Ape into Man: A Study of Human Evolution. Boston, MA: Little, Brown, 1974.

White R. Motivation reconsidered: the concept of competence. Psychological Review 1959; 66: 297–332.

Wolfson WE. American Indian Utensils: Make Your Own Baskets, Pottery and Woodenware with Natural Materials. New York, NY: CIP McKay, 1979.

Ziker JP. Assigned territories: family, clan, communal holdings and common pool resources in the Tarimyr autonomous region, Northern Russia. Human Ecology: An Interdisciplinary Journal 2003; 31: 331–68.

CHAPTER 4

The therapeutic benefits of creativity

JENNIFER CREEK

Introduction

Since the time of the ancient Greeks and Romans, the relationship between what people do and the state of their health has been recognized (Wilcock, 2001). Some forms of occupation, such as unremitting, hard, physical labour in unpleasant or unsafe surroundings, are known to damage health. On the other hand, involvement in a balanced range of different activities can lead to harmony and balance of body and mind (Wilcock, 2001).

An understanding of how health can be influenced by occupation has led, at certain periods of history, to activities being used for the purposes of therapy. For example, the Roman physician, Galen, recommended treating mental disorders with 'travel, occupational therapy and, for the educated, an increasing participation in lectures, discussions, reading and in pastime creative activities' (Seigel, 1973; as cited in Paterson, 2002, p. 4). In nineteenth-century Scotland, craft activities, such as spinning, knitting, basketry and sewing, were used in the lunatic asylums for therapeutic purposes, along with gardening, singing, dancing and reading (Groundes-Peace, 1957). It was claimed that, 'nothing contributes so much to promote a cure and prevent a relapse' (Groundes-Peace, 1957, p. 17).

In the twentieth century, ideas about the importance of various forms of activity to health led to the development of specialized forms of treatment that became the province of different healthcare professions. These include occupational therapists, music therapists, drama therapists, dance and movement therapists, and art therapists. All these groups employ creative activities for the purposes of maintaining or improving health, although they may work from different philosophical and theoretical bases.

Occupational therapists, for example, are concerned with 'the meaning and purpose that people place on occupations and activities and on the impact of illness, disability, social deprivation or economic deprivation on their ability to carry out those occupations and activities' (Creek, 2003, p. 56). The types of activities used as therapeutic media by occupational therapists include 'art and craft activities, creative activities, self-care activities, work activities, leisure activities, lifestyle activities (such as gardening or routine walking), community outings or social activities' (Creek, 2003, p. 41). It can be seen that occupational therapists use a wide range of activities in therapy, in addition to creative activities.

Other arts therapy professions may be more specialized. For example, art therapists are concerned with assisting clients to produce images or visual representations that express their feelings and to reflect on them: 'The overall aim . . . is to enable a client to effect change and growth on a personal level through the use of art materials in a safe and facilitating environment' (British Association of Art Therapists, 2004).

One of the essential features that all the arts therapies have in common is the use of creative media. In the case of art therapy the medium may be, for example, paint, clay, chalk or pencils, media which allow participants to make an external representation of internal feelings and processes. In drama therapy or dance and movement therapy, the creative medium is the human body. In music therapy, it is the voice and other instruments. Each medium has its own qualities that contribute to the therapeutic process and experience. The use of an expressive medium means that therapy becomes an interaction between four elements: the client, the therapist, the medium and the environment.

Arts and creative activities are widely used for the purposes of therapy in the twenty-first century. This chapter will consider the nature of creativity as it relates to health. Theories of the relationship between creativity and health will be reviewed, drawing conclusions about the mechanisms by which creativity can influence health. Four approaches to therapy, using creative activities, will be described, with examples of some creative-arts-for-health projects.

Relationship between creativity and health

Health has been described as a 'symbolic category . . . of experience that reveals tacit assumptions about individual and social reality . . . Health is a "key word", a generative concept, a value attached to or suggestive of other cardinal values' (Crawford, 1993, p. 133). It is, therefore, not surprising that different groups of people might define *health* in terms that fit with their own values and concerns.

Occupational therapists, for example, often work with people experiencing chronic ill-health or disability, and have defined *health* as 'a dynamic, functional state which enables the individual to perform her or his daily occupations to a satisfying and effective level and to respond positively to change by adapting activities to meet changing needs' (Creek, 2003, p. 54). This definition incorporates the idea that health has a function or practical value.

Health is not an all-or-nothing state but can vary according to circumstances; someone might be healthy in one situation and unhealthy in another. For example, Jane has chronic sarcoidosis, a lung disease that causes progressive breathlessness. She is usually able to carry out all her normal household chores but windy weather increases her breathlessness so that she is unable to do the shopping. If we define health in terms of function, Jane becomes less healthy in windy weather.

Therapists are concerned with improving health and, thus, improving the individual's capacity to function. Those groups of therapists such as art therapists and drama therapists, who use creative activities as therapeutic media, are able to theorize about the relationship between creativity and health in ways that allow them to facilitate the client's movement from a state of ill-health towards a state of positive health and well-being.

Tengland (2001) explored the relationship between creativity and health from a philosophical perspective and concluded that creativity is not necessary within an individual in order to reach acceptable mental health. If, as Tengland suggested, creativity is needed to solve the problems of daily life, we can benefit from the creativity of others. For example, if my neighbour gives me an exotic vegetable from his allotment, I do not have to invent a way to cook it but can find a recipe in a cookery book.

The Russian psychologist, Vygotsky (1994), took the opposite point of view, seeing creativity as an essential human attribute. Creativity underpins the ability to imagine situations and events that are not present and actual. This ability frees our behaviour, thinking, perception and action from dependence on real situations and subservience to the stimuli that happen to be present. Vygotsky (1994) asserted that:

> imagination and creativity are linked to a free reworking of various elements of experience, freely combined, and which, as a precondition, without fail, require the level of inner freedom of thought, action and cognizing which only he who has mastered thinking in concepts can achieve. (Vygotsky, 1994, p. 269)

Someone who loses the capacity for creative thought, perhaps due to brain injury, loses the ability to choose how to act.

The definition of health given above, and adopted by the UK College of Occupational Therapists, incorporates the ability 'to respond positively to change by adapting activities to meet changing needs' (Creek, 2003,

p. 54). If, as Vygotsky suggested, creativity is a necessary component of volitional action, then absence of creativity will mean an inability to adapt activities for particular ends and, hence, failure to maintain health.

The South African occupational therapist, du Toit (1974, p. 87; as cited by du Toit, 1991), suggested that creative ability is a 'combination of an inner volition or drive towards action, and the externalisation or expression of that volition in action'. The individual uses imagination to visualize a desired end and to determine a course of action to achieve that end. For example, if I wish to get fitter, I can imagine various ways of doing so, such as joining a gym, going swimming regularly, taking dance classes or buying an exercise video. I then exercise my volition in choosing which of these activities to take up.

Three psychological elements underpin creative ability: knowledge and skills; creativity facilitating abilities (such as the ability to make new connections and branch out from what is known); and motivation (Necka, 1986; as cited in Cropley, 1997). Each of these elements influences the extent to which we are able to make creative decisions and act on them. For example, in order to choose actions that will support or improve health, individuals need to have knowledge of what those actions might be and the skills to carry them out. In addition, they have to have the drive to carry out their chosen activities. The ability to think creatively and branch out from what is known comes into play when there are barriers or obstacles in the way. The more able individuals are to think creatively, the more likely they are to find ways round the obstacles.

Deficiencies in any of the three elements of creative ability can lead to problems in carrying out creative activities and, hence, can affect health. Therapeutic interventions may be targeted at any or all of them: increasing knowledge and skills; encouraging flexibility of thought and action; and developing motivation and volition.

The different ways of thinking about the relationship between creativity and health outlined above have led to a variety of approaches to using the arts as therapy. Four distinct schools of thought can be identified:

- Creative activities can be applied as a form of psychotherapy. For example, when used as a projective technique, art produces an external image of internal, unconscious feelings, conflicts and processes. This material from the unconscious mind thus becomes more accessible to exploration and change.
- Creative activities allow for the expression of feelings without the use of language. In expressive arts therapy, the art process and the art product are themselves change processes.
- Play is used extensively as therapy with children but playfulness is also an aspect of some therapies for adults. For example, the spontaneity

and transience of the movements made in dance movement therapy require a playful approach on the part of both therapist and client (Payne, 1992).

• In recent years, much work has been done on the effects of creative activity on health, particularly mental health. This has led to the use of creative activities for the purposes of mental health promotion. This topic is covered in more detail in Chapter 9, but an example of a mental health promotion project will be given here.

Each of these four approaches will now be discussed in more detail, with examples of their application.

Creative activities as psychotherapy

The creative process is usually described as taking place in four stages (*see* Chapter 2). The second stage of this process is called 'incubation' and is when the individual, having recognised that a problem does not have an immediate or obvious solution, puts it to one side and does not consciously think about it. During this stage, the mind continues to work on the problem at an unconscious or preconscious level, retrieving relevant information and putting it together in new patterns and perceptions.

Koestler (1974; cited in Flach, 1980) described thought processes during this stage as taking place on more than one level of consciousness. This means that there is a relaxation of the 'controls that normally characterize logical thought processes' (Flach, 1980, p. 511), allowing the emergence of more primitive ways of thinking and feeling. For this relaxation to take place, it is necessary to be able to think in a flexible way, without undue anxiety.

Arts therapists use creative media to assist their clients to get in touch with material from different levels of consciousness within the relative safety of an activity, such as painting or drama. Fidler and Fidler (1963, p. 81) made the point that, 'Those ideas, attitudes, and emotions that are acted out are much less likely to come under the scrutiny of one's more conscious intellectual repressing mechanisms. For this reason, the action of the patient is quite likely to reveal more of the unconscious'.

In psychoanalysis, the ego defence mechanism of projection is used to explore and give insight into the personality. Projection 'involves the individual investing another person [or thing] with qualities that are either desired or, more commonly, unacceptable within the self' (Thompson and Blair, 1998, p. 53). When a creative medium is used for projection, such as a lump of clay, the resulting object can be discussed so that the client is able to talk about his unacceptable qualities as though they were separate from the self and, in theory, increase his self-awareness in a non-confrontational way. Blair (1996; as cited in Thompson and Blair, 1998) felt that projective techniques can be very powerful tools for exploring deep levels of the mind and, hence, can be distressing for the client. She emphasized the importance of balancing explorative work with more ego-supportive techniques, and of using group dynamics to support individuals.

Fidler and Fidler (1963) believed that creative activities could be used for working through unconscious conflicts and building a realistic self-concept. This may be done with or without discussion of the issues and process. Fidler and Fidler (1963, p. 83) described how creative activities could provide the kind of experiences that lead to 'the realistic growing awareness of one's inner self (ego) as well as of body concepts'. These experiences include:

> moving the body in a dance or circle game in response to sound, rhythm, or feeling; communicating with another person, experiencing physical contact, touching and identifying parts of one's own body; acting out feelings in a play; tracing a body or head; reproducing a still life from one's perceptions; creating from a lump of clay or an assortment of paints. (Fidler and Fidler, 1963, p. 84)

The 'Dancing for Living' project is an example of a creative activity, carried out by women with mental health problems, that led to changes in their ways of coping with difficult feelings and in their self-concept.

Dancing for Living

The 'Dancing for Living' project was part of a programme of research exploring alternatives to psychiatric approaches to coping and living with mental distress (Cook et al., 2003). The research team was made up of three women who had all used mental health services themselves, and the project investigated the effects of '5 Rhythms' dancing on women's mental and emotional well-being.

'5 Rhythms' dancing is:

> a system of free dance that allows everyone to discover and enjoy their own 'inner dancer'. There are no steps to learn, and anyone can do it no matter what their age, shape or level of fitness . . . The 5 Rhythms are a kind of map that encourages you to explore different ways of being in movement naturally. They can be seen as the rhythms in which we live our lives. We call them flowing, staccato, chaos, lyrical and stillness. Together they form an energy wave, so the dance is sometimes called 'wave dancing'. (Greenhill, 2003; as cited in Cook et al., 2003, p. 27)

The research team advertised in a local magazine for women to volunteer to come to four dance workshops and to take part in the research.

Volunteers were also found through local networks, such as local '5 Rhythms' dance groups. Twenty participants attended the first workshop and 18 completed the research. Data were collected from several different sources, including:

• diaries kept by the participants, in which they could write or draw anything they felt relevant to the research
• a questionnaire about the women's characteristics and opinions on what makes dance sessions accessible
• peer interviews about the experience of dancing
• three focus groups exploring the effects of the dance on emotional well-being and emotional health
• group discussion of the draft report.

Overall, participants found the experience of '5 Rhythms' dance very enjoyable and positive. They identified three main ways in which the dance had a beneficial effect on their mental and emotional health. First, they felt that the dance helped them to move from feeling stuck to experiencing a flow of energy and a wide range of emotions. Second, the dance released powerful feelings that may have been blocked for a long time. Third, there was a sense of integrating parts of the self, such as self-awareness, spirituality and creativity.

The effects of the dance carried over into everyday life in positive ways. For example, the physical exercise benefited physical health and encouraged participants to take better care of their bodies. Participants also felt that their mental and emotional well-being improved in various ways, from dealing with bottled up feelings to building self-confidence. One woman contrasted the 'quick fix' offered by medication with the movement through fear that took place through dance (Cook et al., 2003, p. 17).

The researchers acknowledged the limitations of such a small piece of research but concluded that their findings add to a growing body of evidence of the beneficial effects of creative arts on general and mental health.

Creative activities as self-expression

Expressing feelings, both positive and painful, is a common and effective way of coping with them. Self-expression is a form of communication, although it may not be directed towards a particular recipient. Fidler (1999) described the process by which:

> the internalized sense of self as an acceptable and valuable human being evolves in part out of and in turn is reflected in one's communication skills and patterns . . . engagement with objects and their related activity provide

opportunities to experiment with ways of relating, connecting, and communicating. (Fidler, 1999, p. 40)

Feelings that are repressed or denied may cause problems to the individual, either through displacement on to unrelated objects, spontaneous expression in inappropriate situations or turning inward on the self. Conversely, appropriate and adequate expression of feelings can lead to a reduction in feelings of stress and a general feeling of well-being.

The American sculptor, J. Seward Johnson, wrote about the importance of using activities to reclaim a basic sense of self through expressing our animal nature because doing so is 'psychologically therapeutic' (Johnson, 1996, p. 24). He related how activities such as painting a picture or lying on one's back in the park and studying the clouds are 'not only expressions of being, these are *declarations of being*' (Johnson, 1996, p. 24).

Creative media can be used by anyone for self-expression but they are especially useful for people who have difficulty with verbal communication. For example, a therapist was asked to work with a small group of young men with learning disabilities living in an institution. All of them had very limited verbal ability, they were all physically fit and they all indulged in serious forms of self-injurious behaviour. The psychiatrist thought that they might benefit from the opportunity to explore and express their feelings through art media. At first, all the men found it difficult to stay in the art room for more than a few minutes, although they usually returned several times during the hour that the session lasted. They were reluctant to use the art materials provided but could be persuaded to paint for short periods of time before losing interest. The therapist alternated painting with listening to brief pieces of music to assist the participants to maintain their interest in the session.

Over a period of about a year, all the participants began to stay in the room for longer periods and concentrate on the activity for more of the time that they were there. During the sessions, there were no attempts at self-harm and there was a dramatic reduction in restless behaviour. Several times, the young men came over to the art room at different times of the week, asking for the group. However, there was no overall reduction in self-injurious behaviour outside the group environment.

Opening shutters – opening minds

'Opening shutters – opening minds' (McKillop, 2003) is an example of a creative arts project that enabled a man with dementia to find a new way of expressing himself. James was diagnosed with dementia after several years of 'wandering in the wilderness' (McKillop, 2003). He had been experiencing depression, confusion and an inability to function, which led to loss of confidence and social isolation. He also wrote that he was 'ostracized from life'. After diagnosis, he came into contact with Alzheimer Scotland Action on Dementia (ASAD) and was put into contact with Marilyn, a skilled photographer. Over a period of several months, she encouraged him to start taking photographs again.

James had previously only taken holiday snaps but, with support and encouragement, he began to relearn how to use a camera. Gradually, he began to develop more confidence and started to use his photographs to try to express moods. The concrete outcome of the project is a book of photographs, with accompanying commentary by James. The main outcomes for James were an increase in confidence through discovering that he could still learn new skills, and a creative medium for expressing himself that released him from being trapped within his condition.

Play and playfulness

Play is difficult to define, not least because it is a personally constructed experience that cannot necessarily be detected by an observer. Someone playing a game of football may have a clear goal and take the activity very seriously, whereas another person engages in the game for pleasure. Both can be seen to be playing but only the second person is approaching the game playfully.

Playfulness involves spontaneity and flexibility in actions and interactions (Knox, 1996). It requires that the player suspend some of the rules of physical and social reality in order to create other possibilities. Children at play will say 'Let's pretend . . .' or 'What if . . .', thus opening up spaces where they can experiment with new ways of behaving and relating. By making explicit that what they are doing is not real, children create situations in which it is safe to imagine alternative versions of reality and try out alternative ways of doing things.

The American occupational therapist Parham (1996) felt that two key features of play are that it is intrinsically motivated and that it is experienced as pleasurable. She claimed that play is health promoting because it involves the experience of pleasure in the here and now. It is 'an expression of our humanity throughout the lifespan [and] an active ingredient of a healthy, satisfying lifestyle' (Parham, 1996, p. 78).

Play is a legitimate activity for children but, despite the assertion that it is important throughout the lifespan, it is often considered less important, or even less acceptable, for adults. Modern Western society is goal-oriented and materialistic, both of which characteristics are not conducive to playfulness. The American occupational therapist Reilly (1974a, p. 68), suggested that play needs to be 'freed from the subservients [sic] to other purposes' because it is, by definition, self-activating and self-rewarding. Indeed, play does not occur in the presence of strong drives that lead to goal-directed behaviour. Play is about fun, joy, flexibility and flow, not about arriving at a particular outcome.

Thompson and Blair (1998) suggested that the creative arts are seen as a legitimate form of play for adults. However, it can also be a challenge for the therapist to move clients from goal-directed behaviour towards finding pleasure in creative activity for its own sake. For example, individuals may not feel safe enough to risk approaching an activity playfully in case the end result is unsatisfactory, or they may be inhibited by anxiety.

Reilly (1974b) proposed that play behaviour is characterized by the exploratory drive of curiosity. It is 'the product of an autonomous capacity to be interested in the environment' (Reilly, 1974b, p. 146), and has a focus on sensory experience. This theory suggests that in order to elicit a playful response from clients, therapists should present activities in ways that trigger their clients' curiosity. For example, a therapist was teaching arts and crafts to primary school children living in conditions of social and economic deprivation, as part of a holiday play scheme. She found that children over the age of eight are very concerned about the opinions of their peers. They want to fit into the social group and are afraid to risk being different. They are therefore much less playful and spontaneous than the younger children. In order to capture the older children's attention and engage their interest in creative activities, the therapist attempted to arouse their curiosity in two ways. First, she designed activities that were challenging so that the children wanted to find out if they could achieve the end product. Second, she offered lots of high quality materials so that the children had a good choice and could explore putting different ones together.

Playful elements of creative activity groups

Participants in two creative activity groups perceived the playful elements of the experience as therapeutic benefits of the activities. Two occupational therapists led an open creative activity group for women with severe, enduring mental illness in a social services day centre. All the women lived in their own homes or in sheltered accommodation, although most of them had interludes in hospital. Each one who was referred to the group was invited to attend for four sessions to see if she found it helpful. She was then able to contract to attend a further eight sessions if she wished to.

In order to evaluate the effects of the group, each woman was interviewed and helped to set personal goals for the group. After eight weeks, each woman was interviewed again to review her goals. During these review interviews, many of the women talked about aspects of the group

that they found helpful. These therapeutic benefits included playful
aspects of the group experience, such as pleasure, flow and flexibility:

'It is fun – you can have a laugh.' (pleasure)

'I like doing something complicated that you can concentrate on. It relaxes
you and takes your mind off your problems.' (flow)

'I started off thinking I wasn't artistic but have been pleased with what I
have achieved.' (flexibility of thought.)

Several participants also commented on the good-humoured interactions
between the two therapists, highlighting these exchanges as one of the
helpful aspects of the group. The playful, relaxed and joyful actions and
interactions of the therapists were seen as a model of how participants
could behave in the group.

One of the occupational therapists also ran a drop-in, creative activity
group for women living in conditions of social and economic deprivation. (This group is described in more detail below.) The effectiveness of
the group was evaluated through a group discussion, facilitated by a visiting therapist. The discussion was recorded. One of the topics discussed
by the women concerned the features of the group that they found helpful; they were similar to the features identified by the first group of
women:

- having a laugh (pleasure)
- concentrating on something takes the mind off worries (flow)
- enjoy learning something new (flexibility).

The features of the two groups identified as helpful by participants are
not only aspects of creativity but they have also been found to support
positive mental health. This will be explored further in the next section.

Creativity and mental health promotion

A range of protective mechanisms and processes have been found to support positive mental health by enabling people to experience stress and
adversity without succumbing to them. Different people are able to with-
stand different levels of stress. These individual variations in vulnerability
are called 'emotional resilience'. The resilient individual is able to maintain positive self-esteem and self-efficacy in the face of adversity and to
manage stress effectively (Rutter, 1987).

Factors that have been found to promote resilience are located in three
domains: personal qualities, the family in which the child grows up, and
the environment (Newman, 2002). The domain on which creative

therapies can have the most direct impact is personal qualities. The characteristics of people who demonstrate high emotional resilience include:

- an easy temperament, active and good-natured
- high intelligence or an aptitude for a particular skill
- good social skills
- personal awareness of strengths and limitations
- feelings of empathy for others
- internal locus of control
- attractiveness to others (Newman, 2002)
- openness to new situations
- sense of humour
- feelings of self-esteem and self-efficacy (Rutter, 1987)
- ability to see order rather than chaos
- a feeling that life makes sense (Antonovsky, 1993).

Mental health promotion projects that employ creative activities as the medium of change are based on the premise that at least some of these characteristics can be developed through the creative process. The Pennywell arts and crafts group illustrates this.

Pennywell arts and crafts group

Pennywell housing estate, in Sunderland, UK, is home to more than 10,500 people, one-third of whom are under the age of 16. It is an area of high unemployment, and is described as suffering from considerable social and economic disadvantage (Pennywell PMS Pilot, 2001). Significant features of the area include high crime rates, poverty, a large number of single-parent families, high levels of ill-health and poor access to effective health and social services.

In 1990, Pennywell Neighbourhood Centre was established through a partnership between local resident groups and various statutory organizations, and funded with Single Regeneration Budget money. The Centre provides a range of social and family support including a nursery, a youth participation project, health education classes and activity sessions for various groups of residents. One of these sessions was a drop-in arts-and-crafts group for women on Monday mornings.

In 2000, the Neighbourhood Centre moved into a new building, sharing it with the local medical centre. Staff running the women's group recognized that many of the participants had mental health needs that were not being met, so they asked the occupational therapist from the medical centre to take over the group. The group then ran for just over a year, with between six and ten participants. The therapist's aims for the group were to:

- offer opportunities to engage in a range of creative activities, with or without an end product
- provide a safe forum for women to explore their own creative potential
- broaden the experience of activity of women with social and/or mental health problems.

The Pennywell Neighbourhood Centre provided a room and a small budget for materials. The women expected to learn a new craft every week and to produce a finished article by the end of the two-hour session. At first, no one was interested in continuing the same project over more than one session, which meant that everyone did the same craft at the same time. After a few months, the occupational therapist began to link projects so that, rather than taking home what they made each week, the women would leave their products at the Centre to work on the following week. For example, they might decorate paper with marbling one week and then use it to cover a notebook the next week.

The original plan was to interview each participant individually, after the group had been running for six weeks, in order to identify personal goals for the groups. However, this plan did not work and it was not possible to make a formal assessment of changes to the women's mental health over the course of the group. Attendance was voluntary, and the women saw the purpose of the group as time out of their difficult daily lives, not as therapy. An attempt to interview individuals to find out what they saw as the benefits of the group failed to elicit any useful information and increased participants' anxiety.

After the failure of the interviews, data about the effects of the group were collected from three sources.

- Attendance records: these showed that about eight women attended the group regularly for periods of several months. Several of them attended regularly for the whole year.
- A group discussion facilitated by a visiting occupational therapist, after the group had been running for about six months.
- Observation and detailed records of each session by the occupational therapist.

The group discussion elicited benefits that the women perceived from attending the group.

- It helped them to structure their time. Participants looked forward to attending the group and thought about it at other times.
- They got pleasure both from the activities and from the company of other group members.

- Their self-esteem was increased through making objects that they were proud of and for which they received praise.
- Concentrating on the activity for two hours and enjoying the company of other participants was relaxing and took their minds off any problems at home.

The therapist observed two major changes in the performance of the women.

- Increased initiative: for the first few months, everyone did the same activity every week. As people became more confident, they began to ask to continue projects, or to take their work forward in different ways.
- Increased self-confidence: at first, everyone would ask for constant guidance and reassurance, and seek help from the therapist immediately if they got into difficulties. Gradually, they began to persist with a task, even when it was not going well, and would try different ways of getting the results they wanted. Several of them would offer to help each other.

It can be seen that these two sets of benefits have much in common with the list of personal characteristics of emotionally resilient individuals.

Summary and conclusion

This chapter has explored the relationship between creativity and health, and has identified groups of healthcare professionals who use that relationship to inform their therapeutic approaches. Four approaches to therapy were outlined: psychotherapy, expressive arts, play and mental health promotion. Examples were given to illustrate how these approaches have been used in clinical practice. Each of these examples highlighted the therapeutic benefits of the creative arts, either from the point of view of the participants or from more formal evaluation.

It can be seen that the potential benefits to health of creative activities are wide-ranging, from giving temporary respite from anxiety to releasing blocked feelings, integrating aspects of the self and building self-confidence. One theme that runs through these accounts is that the therapeutic use of creative arts is experienced as powerful yet safe and non-intrusive. Creative expression breaks down barriers within the mind, whereas the structure of the activity contains participants in a supportive way.

There has been some research into all four therapeutic approaches, but much more is needed if the creative arts are to become a serious challenge to more traditional medical and psychological therapies.

A review of some of the research that has been done to date can be found in Chapters 5 and 6.

References

Antonovsky A. The sense of coherence as a determinant of health. In: Beattie A, Gott M, Jones J, Sidell E (eds), Health and Well-being: A Reader. Basingstoke: Macmillan, 1993; 202–11.

British Association of Art Therapists (2004). (Accessed 18 March 2004: www.baat.org/art_therapy.html)

Cook S, Ledger K, Scott N. Dancing for Living: Women's Experience of 5 Rhythms Dance and the Effects on their Emotional Well-being. Sheffield: UK Advocacy Network, 2003.

Crawford R. A cultural account of 'health': control, release and the social body. In: Beattie A, Gott M, Jones L, Sidell M (eds), Health and Well-being: A Reader. Basingstoke: Macmillan, 1993; 113–43.

Creek J. Occupational Therapy Defined as a Complex Intervention. London: College of Occupational Therapists, 2003.

Cropley AJ. Creativity and mental health in everyday life. In: Runco MA, Richards R (eds), Eminent Creativity, Everyday Creativity and Health. Greenwich, CT: Ablex, 1997; 231–46.

Fidler GS. The language of objects. In: Fidler GS, Velde BP (eds), Activities: Reality and Symbol. Thorofare, NJ: Slack, 1999; 37–45.

Fidler GS, Fidler JW. Occupational Therapy: A Communication Process in Psychiatry. New York, NY: Macmillan, 1963.

Flach FF. Psychobiologic resilience, psychotherapy and the creative process. Comprehensive Psychiatry 1980; 21: 510–18.

Groundes-Peace ZC. An outline of the development of occupational therapy in Scotland. Scottish Journal of Occupational Therapy 1957; 30: 16–39.

Johnson JS. Realistic expression: statements of being. In: Zemke R, Clarke F (eds), Occupational Science: The Evolving Discipline. Philadelphia, PA: FA Davis, 1996; 23–5.

Knox SH. Play and playfulness in preschool children. In: Zemke R, Clarke F (eds). Occupational Science: The Evolving Discipline. Philadelphia, PA: FA Davis, 1996; 81–8.

McKillop J. Opening Shutters – Opening Minds. Stirling, Scotland: Dementia Services Development Centre, 2003.

Newman T. Promoting Resilience: A Review of Effective Strategies for Child-care Services. Exeter, England: Centre for Evidence Based Social Services, University of Exeter, 2002.

Parham LD. Perspectives on play. In: Zemke R, Clarke F (eds). Occupational Science: The Evolving Discipline. Philadelphia, PA: FA Davis, 1996; 71–80.

Paterson CF. A short history of occupational therapy in psychiatry. In: Creek J (ed.), Occupational Therapy and Mental Health (third edition). Edinburgh: Churchill Livingstone, 2002; 3–14.

Payne H. Introduction. In: Payne H (ed.), Dance Movement Therapy: Theory and Practice. London: Routledge, 1992; 1–17.

Pennywell PMS Pilot. The Pennywell PMS Pilot: An Evaluation Report. Sunderland, England: Pennywell Medical Centre, Portsmouth Road, Pennywell, 2001.

Reilly M. An explanation of play. In: Reilly M (ed.), Play as Exploratory Learning: Studies of Curiosity Behaviour. Beverly Hills, CA: Sage, 1974a; 117–149.

Reilly M. Defining a cobweb. In: Reilly M (ed.), Play as Exploratory Learning: Studies of Curiosity Behaviour. Beverly Hills, CA: Sage, 1974b; 57–116.

Rutter M. Psychosocial resilience and protective mechanisms. American Journal of Orthopsychiatry 1987; 57: 316–31.

Tengland P. Mental Health: A Philosophical Analysis. Dordrecht: Kluwer Academic, 2001.

Thompson M, Blair SEE. Creative arts in occupational therapy: ancient history or contemporary practice? Occupational Therapy International 1998; 5: 49–65.

du Toit V. Patient Volition and Action in Occupational Therapy. Hillbrow, South Africa: Vona and Marie du Toit Foundation, 1991.

Vygotsky L. Imagination and creativity of the adolescent. In: van der Veer R, Valsiner J (eds), The Vygotsky Reader. Oxford: Blackwell, 1994; 266–88.

Wilcock AA. Occupation for Health, Volume 1: A Journey from Self Health to Prescription. London: College of Occupational Therapists, 2001.

CHAPTER 5

Factors that encourage or inhibit creativity: current and new directions for research

FRANCES REYNOLDS

Introduction

The complex interplay between creativity and health can be explored in many ways. Many issues have been addressed by researchers, such as whether creativity is confined to those with extraordinary personality traits and cognitive abilities or whether it should be regarded as a universal human trait or capability. Is an individual's level of creativity fixed at an enduring level or does it fluctuate according to situational context and life events? Are there gender differences in creativity? Personal, social and developmental issues have dominated the attention of researchers in this field (Simonton, 2000) and these issues will be explored in this chapter. The question of whether people's engagement in creativity influences their psychological and physical health has been given much less research attention, and the evidence will be discussed in a subsequent chapter. In the context of public health, it is important to find out whether only an élite minority manifests creativity, because this would suggest that creative occupations have limited general relevance for promoting health and well-being. If, on the other hand, research confirms that creativity is a universal human attribute, open to discovery and resurgence in certain supportive social contexts, then the case for promoting public health through creative opportunities will be strengthened.

This chapter will review studies that have addressed the following questions:

- Are certain personal and social characteristics associated with creativity?
- Are particular individuals more creative than others by virtue of personality and psychological health, gender or other traits and characteristics?
- Is creativity affected by ageing?
- How do changes in mental and physical health influence creativity?

90

• Can creativity be released by illness; for example, in certain circumstances, do adverse life events encourage people to adopt a more self-actualizing lifestyle?

It is inevitable that only a selection of research studies can be considered in the space of one chapter. This review focuses mainly on research on adult creativity published since 1990, and attempts to acquaint the reader with a wide array of research methods. Psychologists have focused particularly on defining and measuring creativity. They have studied whether certain personality and intellectual characteristics encourage creativity and focused on identifying relevant contextual influences (Simonton, 2000). The chapter will present a number of suggestions for taking research in this field in new directions. As a result, the reader may be encouraged to carry out further research into the factors that encourage creativity and the benefits of creativity for health and well-being. Such research is needed to develop the evidence-base for health promotion interventions.

Defining and assessing creativity

How should we define and assess creativity? Agreement on these issues would seem to be vital if valid research is to be carried out. However, as we will see in this chapter, researchers are far from achieving consensus about their subject matter and use a wide variety of assessment tools and research methods.

Creativity as traits or behaviours

Some investigators have defined creativity in terms of certain individual traits or behaviours, in particular originality (unusual or unexpected responses), fluency or productivity (focusing on quantity and sometimes rapidity of responses) and usefulness (value or appropriateness within the context), as outlined by Cooper (1991). Other attributes of the creative individual have been shown to include openness to experience, abstraction, resistance to premature closure, and tolerance of ambiguity (Amabile, 1990; Orwoll and Kelley, 1998). A number of pencil-and-paper cognitive tests have been developed to assess these characteristics. For example, the Torrance Tests provide subtests that measure a number of the traits outlined above, and the Barron–Welsh Art Scale assesses individuals' preferences for visual stimuli that differ in symmetry, ambiguity and complexity (Cooper, 1991). These types of creativity test appear to assume that creativity is an enduring intellectual trait within the person, rather than a function of the interactions between the individual and the wider context (a systems approach).

Psychological tests also tend to assume that creativity is context-independent. That is, they underplay the possibility that the individual's creativity varies according to the domain of the activity and its social context. For example, a person who engages in writing poetry may not be so creative when painting. People's level of creativity may also depend on whether they are familiar with the media being presented, their level of expertise, and the broader context (for example, whether the social environment is competitive or supportive). 'Real world' creativity does seem to depend upon having a certain level of expertise (Lubart and Sternberg, 1998). As a further problem, some pencil-and-paper creativity tests are limited because they assess divergent thinking only, whereas real-world problem-solving (and most scientific and artistic work) generally requires cycles of divergent and convergent thinking to achieve a skilful and appropriate outcome (Brown, 1989).

Although many tests show adequate reliability, in that individuals score fairly consistently over time, there is evidence that creativity tests may not measure what they claim to measure. In other words, such tests may lack validity. Cooper (1991) examined six pencil-and-paper creativity tests and showed that, in some tests, the scoring system simply reflects the quantity or fluency of individuals' responses within a given period of time rather than their quality. Some test items seem to reflect very narrow conceptualizations of creativity. For example, the Structure of Intellect Learning Abilities Test assesses creativity in terms of how many small squares the respondent can fill with drawings taken from different categories of object (*see* Cooper, 1991). These responses require little skill and limited lateral thinking. The respondent may even lose points simply from not guessing what kinds of responses are being valued by the researcher's scoring system.

The design of the test material itself is crowded and distracting, inhibiting deep engagement with the subject matter. Such problems with visual crowding occur in other tests also, such as the Torrance Test of Creative Thinking. Cooper (1991, p. 202) also argued that some tests seem to be 'looking for a goody-goody, supremely well adjusted type of creative person', overlooking the possibility that negative emotional and personality traits may heighten creative self-expression in some circumstances (Schuldberg, 1990; Helson, 1999). Furthermore, creativity testing seems to ignore the everyday observation that creative individuals often flourish in one particular domain only (for example, musical performance, scientific enquiry, mechanical invention). It is unclear whether the same intellectual, emotional and personality attributes underpin all these diverse abilities.

Creativity as eminence

Some investigators have preferred to define creativity in terms of public acclaim or eminence. Albert (1990, p. 14) saw creative people as having 'achieved recognition and ranking by others who are expert and experienced enough to appreciate and judge particular performances and results'. It is this view that led Csikszentmihalyi (1990) to argue that creativity cannot be regarded simply as the property of individuals. He represented it instead as the attribute of 'social systems making judgements about individuals' (Csikszentmihalyi, 1990, p. 198). Researchers who have accepted this definition have focused their enquiries on the personality traits and other enabling characteristics of eminent practitioners, such as famous artists, musicians, scientists and architects. As an inevitable consequence, their findings and theorizing about creative processes and outcomes inevitably relate to a highly selected, élite group within the population.

Research that defines creativity in terms of what is considered highly original and useful by outsiders has the unfortunate effect of excluding more everyday forms of creativity from view. Everyday or practical creativity includes successful problem-solving in daily situations, and dealing with ambiguity (Marsiske and Willis, 1998). It is manifested in tasks as diverse as preparing aesthetic, nutritious and tasty meals on a low budget, beautifying our home environment and inventing stories at bedtime for our children. As all these activities involve at least some innovation and originality, they may be considered creative. Their role in enhancing satisfaction with life, self-esteem and a sense of self-efficacy certainly seems worthy of study. Yet, creativity researchers have largely neglected these forms of creative behaviour.

Creativity as intrinsic motivation

The phenomenological experience offers another facet of creativity to study. Some researchers have chosen to explore people's intrinsic motivation – their interest, enjoyment and satisfaction with the process for its own sake – as the hallmark of creativity (Amabile, 1990). Gedo (1990, p. 35), for example, defined creativity as 'the healthy enjoyment of the search for novelty'. Smith et al. (2002, p. 158) also added a process perspective, stating that creativity is 'a generative or productive way of shaping our conception of reality, including our own selves'. They argued that the creative person enjoys 'open communication among different layers of his or her experiential world' (Smith et al., 2002, p. 158). Researchers who wish to understand more about the creative experience and its psychological benefits have tended to adopt qualitative methods, such as interviews.

Although creativity research has been guided by a plethora of conceptual perspectives, it has, arguably, focused on very small subsets of the human population. The cognitive testing tradition within creativity research has tended to focus disproportionately on school children and undergraduate samples, partly because these are available in large numbers and are convenient for researchers to access. However, such samples do not provide a good microcosm of the wider population, as they are young, many are highly educated, and all have yet to embark on their careers and family responsibilities. It is therefore difficult to decide whether those who score highly on creativity tests are really more creative in their meaningful work and leisure activities as they have had few opportunities to demonstrate this in their everyday lives. From a public health perspective, we may be particularly interested in the creative potential of chronically ill, disabled, and older groups of people. Research that has been over-reliant on undergraduate samples and pencil-and-paper creativity tests arguably has limited power to address this issue.

Research that has defined creativity in terms of public eminence has inevitably selected people for study who are at the peak of their creative careers. This research tradition has thereby excluded from view the creative potential of adults in general and has focused attention on creative *work* rather than *leisure* activities. Simonton (2000, 2002) has pointed out that women and people from ethnic minorities have been particularly under-researched populations in creativity research. We should add chronically ill, disabled and socially disadvantaged people to this list. Researchers urgently need to explore how health and social problems affect everyday creativity, and whether creative endeavour enhances well-being, coping and self-esteem among people living with different forms of physical, psychological and social adversity.

The remainder of the chapter explores research into the personal and social factors that appear to enhance creativity. Chapter 6 examines the influence of creative occupation on physical and psychosocial well-being.

Are certain personal and social characteristics associated with creativity? Research frameworks

What are the precursors of creative behaviour? Are some individuals highly creative throughout their lives or does creativity fluctuate over the life course according to life events, responsibilities, adversities and other experiences? Do highly creative people share certain defining personality traits? Do individuals require high levels of physical and mental well-being in order to be creative, or is this form of activity equally open to people with mental and physical health problems? Does creativity change with ageing, and if so, how? What social forces encourage creativity? All of these questions are relevant to health promotion and public health initiatives, as we need to establish whether creativity is the province of an élite few, or open to all, and whether there might be barriers to engaging in creative activities in later life or during adverse life events.

Three major research frameworks have been used to address this broad set of questions about the origins and impetus of creativity. These include: longitudinal studies of highly creative individuals; cohort studies in which the creativity of people of different ages is assessed quantitatively and compared; and psychoanalytic and other interpretive case studies of eminent artists and other creative individuals. The fourth, but least adopted, framework is broadly phenomenological, asking people who engage in creative activities at various levels of expertise to reflect on the origins of their creative interests and abilities.

Longitudinal studies

Longitudinal studies follow the same individuals, over an extended period, to detect whether they show consistencies or fluctuations in their creative functioning. For example, Dudek and Croteau (1998) and Dudek and Hall (1991) reported a 25-year longitudinal study of eminent architects. Helson and colleagues reported on a longitudinal study of highly creative women, followed up from the age of about 21 to 52 years (Helson, 1990, 1998, 1999; Helson and Pals, 2000; Helson et al., 1995). The longitudinal research design enables individual change and consistency in creativity to be tracked in some detail over the lifespan. Nevertheless, it is an expensive and time-consuming approach to research, requiring extensive funding and a long term commitment from all involved. The findings may also be limited by the original research assumptions and the measures selected at the start, which inevitably reflect the specific intellectual culture of the time. In all longitudinal research, reduction in sample size, due to declining interest of the participants, loss of contact, death and other factors, can jeopardize the validity of the study.

To give one example, the Mills College study was started in the late 1950s to explore the long term development of 30 women students who were judged by college staff as having high creative potential (Helson, 1998). The top 15% of the senior year were nominated, and their siblings and parents also joined the study. They were compared with a group considered low in creative potential but matched in terms of scholastic attainment and academic subjects studied. Large batteries of creative tests, projective tests and personality inventories were administered, and the women's personal characteristics were assessed through in-depth interviews by 'judges' who were blind to the participants' nomination (as high/low creative). The assessments were repeated when the women were 28, 43 and 52 years old, and participants' career progression was monitored.

The study revealed that the women who scored highly on creativity tests tended to be open to experience, tolerant of ambiguity, willing to take risks and able to value their difference from others. They recalled enjoying more creative play activities in childhood, and their parents saw them as head-strong and unconventional, implying that their creativity was a long-standing personal attribute from childhood onwards. Ultimately, they demonstrated higher levels of creativity in their careers than the group considered as having less creative potential (Lubart and Sternberg, 1998).

However, social context was also found to exert an important influence over whether the women fulfilled their creative potential in their subsequent careers. For example, the social role obligation to be a good mother made it difficult for some women to fulfil their creative potential. Gender discrimination also played a role in limiting career progression. Helson noted that women who were successful in their careers at 45 years old tended to lack brothers and, perhaps for this reason, seemed to be regarded as special in their families. Their favoured position within the family possibly helped them to overcome the traditional roles ascribed to daughters in 1950s and 1960s American society. Where present, brothers may have drawn family attention and support away from the women. Helson also noted that the women tended to excel only in certain careers (for example, psychoanalysis, anthropology, social history) where female participation was viewed favourably within the wider culture rather than being seen as a liability.

This longitudinal study is also interesting in showing that creative women do not necessarily have optimally functioning personalities. Some had unresolved identity problems and those specializing in the creative arts in particular, tended to experience more negative emotionality (Helson, 1999). However, Helson and Pals (2000) suggested that creative work might have an integrative influence. Possibly it serves to channel negative emotion in productive directions. Although longitudinal studies have emphasized certain individual consistencies in creative personality and productivity, data analysis also reveals that individuals show certain fluctuations in their creativity according to their social context. For example, women's (and perhaps men's) creativity may vary according to whether they are living in a stable marriage or going through a divorce, and whether or not they achieve a sufficient income from their creative work.

At first sight, the Mills College study seems to imply that creativity is the province of the fortunate few. Yet, even if taken at face value, this evidence – that creative people have distinguishing personality and cognitive attributes from an early age – might imply a need for better nurturance of children's creative potential within the educational system. People perhaps need to be encouraged to think unconventionally and to be self-expressive from pre-school and school days onwards. It is certainly possible that relevant cognitive skills, such as flexibility and tolerance for ambiguity, will only flourish in supportive environments that maintain children's confidence in their self-worth and personal viewpoint. It is also possible that a larger proportion of people would recognize and use the creative potential that they have if they enjoyed greater opportunity and support for creativity within the community context.

Longitudinal studies have illuminated the fascinating trajectory of the lives of creative people as they have unfolded during the last 50 years or so. Yet, the findings need to be evaluated in the context of the specific historical and cultural period in which the participants lived. Also, studies are limited by the suppositions made at their outset, namely, that highly creative people could be identified while at college through quantitative tests and other personality assessments. In the Mills College study, we may also question the creativity ratings that were applied to the women's subsequent careers. For example, teaching received a lower creativity rating than journalism. When we consider how flexible a teacher needs to be, if she is going to be responsive to the changing needs and interests of her classes, we may question the validity of such a rating scale. Furthermore, the reliance on summative, quantitative measures of creativity, personality traits and so on, makes it difficult to understand the complex interplay of personality, intellectual and social factors that shape the creativity of individuals. To gain further insights into developmental trajectories, more research is needed into women's and men's own narrative accounts of growing up in families and schools that nurtured or inhibited creativity.

As the previous discussion has shown, longitudinal studies have focused upon eminent people selected relatively early in life. Such studies tend to emphasize continuities in individual creativity. Cross-sectional, cohort research has provided an alternative means of documenting whether creativity persists, declines or increases during the life course, by comparing groups of people of different ages.

Cohort studies investigating changes in creativity with age

Another issue relevant to understanding the origins of creativity is whether creativity alters with ageing and health problems. Simonton (1975, 1988,

1990, 1998) carried out a number of cohort studies in which the creative output of people of different ages was compared using historiometric methods. By focusing on the creative outputs of selected eminent people, rather than assessing personality and other psychological factors, the data have the advantage of being objective and less open to debate. Such evidence helps to answer the question (commonly posed within the creativity research literature) of whether creativity declines with age.

Simonton's (1975, 1988) earlier work examined the published work of eminent creative people and found evidence of declining productivity in the older age groups. This age-related decline was more marked in some domains of work than others. For example, in 1975, Simonton reported that poets were relatively young when they produced the work for which they would later become famous. However, he noted many exceptions, and has argued in his more recent work that creativity can be maintained in later life by maintaining intellectual contact with colleagues and by re-tooling (Simonton, 1990, 1998). This means continually re-equipping ourselves with new skills and fresh creative interests. On the basis of Simonton's work and other studies, Lubart and Sternberg (1998) put forward the investment theory of creativity, which posits that people's creativity reflects a number of resources – cognitive, affective and social-environmental. They argued that older people may be able to maintain or even extend their creativity, as long as such resources are kept in place through social and intellectual stimulation. It is even possible that by taking up new social and intellectual activities, older people could *enhance* their creativity.

Cohort studies have tended to focus on the rise and fall in creativity over the lifespan, whereas longitudinal studies have emphasized individual continuity and preservation of creative activity, at least among gifted samples. This disparity points to the influence of the specific research question and methodology on research findings. Recent opinion seems to be resolving this disparity by becoming less negative about the creativity of older people (Lindauer, 1998a; Simonton, 1998, 2000). Indeed, Lindauer (1998b) reported on a cohort study in which people in their 20s, 40s, 60s and 80s described their engagement in creative pursuits such as playing musical instruments, visiting museums and art galleries, and painting. There was little sign of decreasing interest in artistic pursuits with age, except among the oldest people who were in the poorest health.

We might ask why some people succeed in maintaining their interests and contextual supports for creative activity in their later years, when others lose them. The answers may be highly relevant to promoting public health. Earlier research generally conceptualized ill-health as removing a person's resources for creativity, but more recent studies have found that illness and disability sometimes result in a positive reappraisal of priorities and self-image, leading to transformational coping among certain individuals (Tedeschi and Calhoun, 1995). This way of coping with adversity may, in turn, be shaped by complex biographical factors and social context. A better understanding of how individuals act creatively within their particular social environments seems most likely to be achieved through case studies, narrative and other qualitative methods, which will be considered next.

Case studies of artists and other creative people

Case studies are based on the intensive, in-depth study of one or a few individuals. Usually, a range of material is brought to bear on the task of understanding the creative motivation of individuals, including evidence about their childhood, their personal values, skills and priorities. These may be ascertained from documents or interviews. Creative output may also be examined for themes, technique and style. The complex case material of clients in psychoanalysis has also been used to formulate theory about the origins of creative motivation. Some retrospective studies, for example the studies by Rodeheaver et al. (1998) and Schwartz (2001), explore the creativity of people who lived long ago, whereas others seek to understand the creativity of living artists.

Clearly, case studies, being naturalistic, offer the potential of gaining insights into the complexity of real-life creativity in ways that pencil-and-paper tests do not. However, because case studies can only be carried out where sufficient documentary material is available, they have tended to focus either on individuals who are eminent in their fields, or on clients engaged in lengthy psychoanalysis. This limits the possibility of generalizing findings to the population at large. Nevertheless, some of these studies do have the advantage of focusing on individuals from neglected populations within creativity research, namely women and disabled people. Also, in their focus on real-world creativity, and in their acceptance of the complexity of lives, such studies arguably carry tentative implications for public health promotion through creative occupation.

A number of case studies and other enquiries have explored the personal and social factors that influence the creativity, specifically, of women. For example, Slatkin (1993) reviewed documents (such as letters and diary accounts) written by a number of acclaimed women artists, to understand the origins of their artistic creativity. The documents mostly revealed these women to have been aware of their artistic potential from an early age. Most had entered formal art training by their late teens. Their families generally offered emotional and financial support for the women's artistic careers, even when not themselves artistically talented.

Strong personal commitment to art and considerable self-belief seemed to energize their work. A supportive social and economic context is often important, especially for women who go on to become artists. The importance of a facilitatory context also emerged in a questionnaire study of 31 female artists by Schwartz (2001). These various findings resonate with those emerging from the longitudinal studies and suggest that, for some individuals, highly creative ability manifests itself early in life. However, the findings challenge the notion of creativity as a consistent personal trait, by emphasizing that adults may not reach their creative potential without family support and mentoring (for example, by teachers) during their formative years. Women, in particular, appear to need encouragement to overcome traditional gender roles and to resist undue social conformity.

Some case studies of creative individuals have sought to establish whether mental health problems motivate creativity, and many of these studies have been framed within a psychoanalytic theoretical perspective (Gedo, 1996, 1997). Given the argument throughout this book, that creative occupation provides an effective means of promoting health and well-being, it may appear contradictory to propose any role for mental health problems in motivating a need for creative expression. Jamison (1993) looked at the self-image, emotional conflicts and behaviours of selected artists, composers and writers, and suggested that many had symptoms of manic-depressive disorder. The manic phase tends to be associated with fluency of ideas and productivity.

Such an analysis is compatible with psychoanalytic theories which propose that creativity and psychopathology have common origins in unconscious defence mechanisms against unbearable anxiety (Domino et al., 2002). Creativity may permit the safe self-expression of unconscious, unacceptable impulses, thereby serving to strengthen the ego, a central component of self. For this reason, some researchers have attempted to understand artistic motivation as sublimating or transforming aggression or sexuality. Day (2002) argued that creativity, in the form of creative writing, is 'a way of confronting anxiety, making peace with one's restorative and destructive effects on the outside world – a process that requires (and builds) ego strength and maturity' (Day, 2002, p. 127). However, there seems to be some debate over whether unresolved conflicts might directly find expression in creative self-expression, or whether some form of therapeutic resolution is first needed. Gedo (1990, p. 37), for example, provided an account of a client who could only embark on writing a novel and poetry when she had completed three years of analysis and had achieved a certain level of well-being. Gedo (1990, p. 37) argued that the client needed to resolve some of her anxieties around being successful before she could 'unleash a great creative talent'. In contrast, he also interpreted another client's creativity as a current strategy to ward off low self-esteem.

This raises the issue of why psychoanalysts interpret 'similar' behaviours in such different ways, and whether this theoretical perspective has validity. We also need to ask whether some psychoanalytic analyses of case material are selective and overinterpretive, and whether or not the explanation for creative behaviour is one that the subjects of the study would agree with. For example, Chave (1990) interpreted the artist Georgia O'Keeffe's striking close-up images of flowers as motivated by unconscious sexual imagery, whereas the artist herself rejected such an explanation, arguing that her work simply revealed a love for the flora of the American landscape. While it remains possible that creative people may erect psychological defences to prevent themselves from recognizing any darker, unconscious meanings within their work, such disputes inevitably raise questions about the validity of psychoanalytic interpretations.

Case studies have illuminated the influences of various positive and negative personality traits, social relationships and adverse events, on creativity. In contrast, research that explores individual continuity across the lifespan, using longitudinal designs, has largely ignored the potential role of crisis, in particular the role of physical illness or mental health problems, in bringing about the discovery (or resurgence) of creativity. Yet 'interrupted and conflicted lives' seem to have a particular potential for creativity (Bateson, 2001, p. 9). Case studies and biographies have shown that certain acclaimed artists have been spurred into art through illness or injury. For example, Frida Kahlo began oil painting while confined to bed during a serious illness (Herrera, 1998). Zausner (1998) examined relationships between physical ill-health and creativity in 21 acclaimed artists and found that about a third had developed their interest in art during periods of long-term illness and convalescence in childhood and adolescence. Such confinement to home (and in many cases to bed) resulted in the experience of unproductive time and the search for a meaningful activity. Illness also confronts the sufferer with issues of self, anxiety and mortality. Some individuals appear to address these deeper concerns through creative self-expression.

Zausner (1998) attempted to explain why artists who had turned to art during illness had selected this activity rather than any other alternative. The presence of artistic adult role models and access to art materials seemed to have been influential. Zausner (1998) also found that some artists had developed their involvement in art only in their later adulthood. Longo-Muth, for example, committed herself to art after retiring from teaching because of multiple sclerosis. She argued that illness is an encouragement 'to direct what energies you have left and focus them on your creativity' (as cited in Zausner, 1998, p. 25).

To conclude, some case study and biographical research has found that ill-health and crisis can be turning points which encourage some individuals to discover and explore their own creativity and artistic skills. This perspective implies that creative occupation may be health-promoting, particularly for individuals facing health problems and other adversities. Nevertheless, we must be cautious about generalizing, as case studies have tended to focus on eminent artists and other highly creative people. Whether the psychological conflicts and life adversities that stimulated their creativity are relevant to the wider population cannot be confidently assumed. Yet, the findings certainly question the assumption, reinforced by several longitudinal studies, that individuals show predictable levels of creativity over the course of their adult lives. Case study research suggests, instead, that crisis events may release previously untapped creative potential depending, of course, upon individuals' own interpretations of these events and their social context. Further research is required to explore whether, and to what extent, people generally respond to adversity with a surge, or loss, of creativity.

As noted above, there has been some research to establish the role of psychopathology in creativity. However, it is not possible from the case study approach to estimate whether psychological problems, such as manic depression, are common in the wider population who enjoy creative occupations. Findings that certain famous artists have coped with manic depression (Jamison, 1993) do not necessarily imply that people generally need to have emotional problems as a prerequisite of creativity. Possibly some artists' personality and emotional difficulties drive their single-minded pursuit of fame and achievement, rather than being responsible for their creativity *per se*. There is no evidence that emotional turmoil is a prerequisite for enjoying more casual, leisure-based creative activities. Furthermore, if we accept the argument that artistic creativity may be motivated by a deep need for self-expression, it is not surprising that people with greater distress or difficulty may have a particular need for the oblique or symbolic self-expression that is permitted by the creative arts (Dekker, 1996). It is also possible that psychological difficulties and psychological health underpin different forms of creative behaviour (Richards, 1990).

More radically, we might question the cultural forces that encourage a search for psychopathology in creative individuals. Becker (2000–2001) argued that the supposed link between madness and creativity is a relatively recent construct within Western culture, originating within the Romantic Movement in the late eighteenth and early nineteenth centuries. It distorts the ancient Greek concept of divine inspiration, and the Renaissance concept of genius, and perhaps suggests a cultural distrust of people regarded as non-conforming or eccentric.

Qualitative and questionnaire studies of people's experiences of creativity

The origins of creativity and creative occupation have also been investigated, in a limited way, through qualitative (often interview-based) studies in which participants are invited to reflect on their own experience. Analysis of the verbal data is conducted through recognized qualitative procedures, such as discourse analysis or grounded theory. Attention is usually given, in the data analysis, to potential researcher bias, which may be controlled by the use of second coders, researcher debriefing and reflection, and consultation with participants about the emergent themes. The analysis of qualitative data may, therefore, achieve an acceptable level of rigour and overcome some of the bias that can be present in more highly interpretive case studies. A few questionnaire studies, for example Christiansen (2000), have also enquired into the personal meanings of hobbies and leisure activities.

Mishler (1999) carried out an in-depth narrative interview study of the lives of five people working in arts and crafts to find out more about their life trajectories as creative individuals. The research revealed the complexity of the artists' lives, and showed that there were both certain consistencies and discontinuities in their creative involvement over time. Some had been committed to art-making from their youth. Others had immersed themselves in their art or craft, or had changed the nature of their art medium in response to an adversity, such as an injury, a divorce or an intensifying feeling of being locked into a stifling small-town environment. The findings emphasized that various contextual factors, including opportunity and support, influence creativity, and that individuals do not necessarily engage in creative work in a consistent fashion. Mishler (1999) argued that we need both theory and more adequate research methods to find out more about such discontinuities in development. While, clearly, we need more information about how and why certain individuals respond to adversity with creative endeavour, the findings provide grounds for optimism that creative opportunities could provide at least some people with a significant means of restoring identity, social connections and hope for the future.

In some cases, the experiences of under-researched groups, such as women, older people and chronically ill people, have been the focus of qualitative enquiry into the origins of creativity and creative occupation. Themes of guilt, role conflict and a 'late start' were discovered in an interview study of factors affecting the productivity of 10 female artists with children (Kirschenbaum and Reis, 1997). Although most of the participants recalled being artistic at school, they had generally received little encouragement to take their studies further. For example, their parents recommended alternative careers with more secure financial prospects, and their husbands were generally unsupportive. Yet, some participants found that they could manage successfully to combine art with their child-care and home responsibilities. Once discovered, art became valued as a means of self-expression. It also provided temporary psychological escapes from the routines of motherhood. However, for many participants, joy mingled with guilt over balancing the roles of wife and mother with that of artist. Research such as this is based on very small self-selected groups and therefore cannot be readily generalized. It is also specific in terms of the participants' historical period and North American culture. Gender roles may have different meanings in other times and places. However, the research was successful in gathering personal accounts that revealed the rich complexity of participants' motivations for art, and it showed how social roles and context might constrain creativity, at least in the case of women. By documenting that some women turn to creative occupations when time and opportunity arise, the study suggests that there are no automatic barriers to taking up creative activities in adulthood. The findings, somewhat reinforced by the longitudinal studies outlined earlier, also challenge élitist notions, that only a small segment of the population is creative and that creative potential is necessarily identifiable in youth or early adulthood.

Lindauer et al. (1997) also argued against the idea that creativity is a prerogative of young people. They surveyed 88 graphic artists aged 60 years and older. According to many of the participants' responses to open-ended questions on a questionnaire, their engagement in art-making increased during their later years, in part because of reduced involvement in alternative activities, such as paid work and family responsibilities, and in part because their artistic skills had developed further (Lindauer, 1998a). They also attributed their creative rejuvenation to a wide range of personality factors, including continuing enthusiasm, openness to experience, commitment to learning and personal growth and self-acceptance. A view of time as precious, and a desire to express an accumulated 'lifetime of emotions' (Lindauer et al., 1997, p. 141) also motivated creative productivity. These motives have been associated with creativity in other studies of older people, for example Fisher and Specht (1999). Participants did not regard their old age and physical limitations as inhibiting their creative work. Indeed, some expressed and perhaps came to terms with these experiences thematically in their artwork (Lindauer, 1998a). Such findings challenge some other studies, for example Lehman (1953), which have reported a decline in creativity with ageing.

As a further example of research examining how illness may stimulate engagement in creative activities, Reynolds (1997, 2000) analysed written accounts by textile artists who were affected by long term physical and mental health problems. Participants described the functions of art in their lives and the experiences that had stimulated their interest in textile arts. More than half of the chronically ill women described taking up art-work after diagnosis, usually to cope with anxiety about the illness or unstructured time, for example, during hospitalization. For some of these women, serendipitous events, such as receiving a needlecraft kit or book, seemed to catalyse their involvement in textile artwork. A later interview-based study found similar results (Reynolds, 2003a; Reynolds and Prior, 2003). Again, these findings suggest that people may have latent creativity that can emerge in later life in response to a number of events. These include the experience of empty time after retirement, or during convalescence, opportunity or invitation, and a reappraisal of life priorities triggered by serious illness. The discovery of textile art as a meaningful occupation, as opposed to other ways of living with illness, appeared to be encouraged by early family role models who enjoyed artwork and sewing, enjoyment of art at school, and the discovery that personal and professional identity could be expressed through artwork (Reynolds, 2003a). Once they had begun creative art-making, participants reported much-improved well-being. This issue will be returned to in Chapter 6.

Some creativity research views creativity as a personal attribute, akin to intelligence or introversion. Psychoanalytic enquiry tends to view creativity as a means of dealing with the individual's inner psyche. However, certain qualitative research studies have discovered that people sometimes take up creative activities for broader social reasons and with a deliberate intention of gaining a better quality of life. For example, Fisher and Specht (1999) interviewed older people who were exhibiting their artwork at a local exhibition and found that their motives for engaging in artwork included enhancing their social status and self-esteem, making friendships and maintaining an active role within the community. Art, for these participants, represented an important way of using time productively, even in the face of their physical limitations. Some of the participants, in an interview study (Reynolds and Prior, 2003), also regarded art-making as a means of living a full and satisfying life in the context of chronic illness. They viewed art as a 'lifestyle coat-hanger' supporting numerous other leisure activities, both intellectual and social (such as visiting museums and taking art classes). This broader conceptualization of the functions and meanings of art-making in people's lives deserves further scrutiny.

Qualitative studies in this area are few. Samples tend to be small and self-selected. It is not possible to generalize about the appeal of creative occupations within the general population from in-depth studies of people who are already committed to art-making or other creative activity. The studies seem to have focused more on women's experience of creativity, leaving men's reasons for practising art and other creative occupations relatively unexplored. Yet, in their favour, we can deduce from these studies that certain people discover creative occupations in their later years, with positive consequences for their health and well-being. Some appear to turn to art-making and other creative pursuits because illness disrupts their regular lifestyles and taken-for-granted priorities; for example, serious ill-health leads to early retirement from work and the appearance of empty time. For some, serious illness provokes critical reflection on existing lifestyle and encourages action to fulfil long-standing aspirations to develop creative talents. For others, creative occupations seem to be taken up primarily to extend social networks during retirement. Creativity may even be discovered through serendipitous events. Such findings seem to suggest that there is much more creative potential in the population at large than earlier researchers assumed, and that creative activities may present a potent, yet neglected, means of promoting health and well-being.

Directions for further research

Although considerable research has been conducted into the personal and social factors that encourage creativity, much remains to be explored. Many issues have been discussed in earlier sections. For example, most of the research focuses on highly selected samples. The longitudinal studies have tended to follow up people initially assessed in their youth as high in creative potential. This approach cannot estimate to what extent creativity is likely to emerge later in adulthood in response to opportunity or adversity. The findings of smaller-scale studies, which have focused on selected cases or on small samples of artists or other creative people, also cannot be confidently generalized to the wider population. Often, samples are necessarily self-selected, as in Reynolds (1997, 2000) and Reynolds and Prior (2003), because the population that engages in artwork as a means of coping with illness is 'hidden' and difficult to sample systematically. A need remains to examine creativity, including motives, skills and achievements, in larger, random samples. Longitudinal designs, in which individuals are tracked over long periods of time, may be helpful for assessing the positive and negative effects of illness, ageing and other changes, on the creative activities of normal adults who are not eminent in the creative sphere.

There is limited evidence that some people respond to the destructuring effects of illness on their daily lives with a heightened commitment to creative occupation. Why some people respond to adverse life events with positive lifestyle change, whereas others feel chronically depressed and demotivated, is an unanswered question. Possibly, larger-scale surveys which include disabled and older people are needed to gain further insights into the personality traits, attitudes and social influences that affect creative self-expression. More in-depth narrative studies could explore people's own interpretations of the creative turning points in their lives. Surveys are also required to determine whether creative opportunities in the community are available, accessible and of interest to disabled people.

Previous research into the roots of creativity has also been inevitably shaped by certain contested definitions of creativity. As long as creativity is assessed by psychometric tests or based on judgements about eminence, everyday creativity will continue to be neglected. Yet, it seems possible that many people value the myriad opportunities that are available for being creative in daily life, albeit in small ways (for example, making a special meal, sewing a cushion cover, planting out a flower tub in the garden). It is unknown whether chronic illness and impairment diminish quality of life through, in part, limiting the possibility of day to day creativity. Conversely, perhaps some individuals protect their wellbeing by taking concerted action to prevent illness from intruding into these everyday creative pursuits. Such issues could be explored, particularly through qualitative methods, in order to gain insights into participants' own experiences of everyday creativity.

Although male participants feature widely in quantitative research based on creativity tests, and in studies of creativity in work organizations, it appears that women have been more extensively studied in qualitative research examining people's motives for creative leisure activities, especially artwork. People from ethnic minorities are greatly under-represented in all creativity research. We need to acknowledge the possible influence of gender and ethnicity on the types of creative occupation that people take up, on the social support that they receive for doing so, and on their willingness to embrace a creative identity in adulthood. There is also a need to explore the effects of mental health on creativity with much more diverse samples than eminent artists and people in psychoanalysis.

Summary and conclusion

Longitudinal studies of people defined in early adulthood as highly creative suggest certain continuities in creative abilities across the lifespan. Case studies, especially those guided by the psychoanalytic perspective, suggest complex (including unconscious) motives for creative self-expression. Some cohort studies challenge the notion that individuals have a consistent level of creative ability, by finding that some individuals experience a resurgence in their creative potential in adulthood. A variety of factors may be responsible for an individual's commitment to creative occupation, including personality traits such as openness to experience, tolerance of ambiguity, coping strategies for dealing with crisis and loss, social roles and opportunity (for example, having free time after retiring from work). However, many forms of research into the origins of creativity tend to be limited both by their restricted focus on the careers and output of highly creative, indeed eminent, participants, and also by their concern with artistic pursuits.

We continue to lack information about the everyday forms of creativity that have great potential to enhance well-being and quality of life. Studies that focus specifically on people defined as highly talented or creative inevitably cannot estimate the creative potential and trajectory of the normal, or indeed adverse, experiences that might spur ordinary people to engage in creative pursuits. The assessment of creativity has tended to be over-reliant on pencil-and-paper creativity testing, career progression or creative work outputs, such as number of cited poems or acclaimed paintings. Such studies do not offer much help in identifying the nurturing social influences that help people to fulfil their creative potential. As a consequence, we have a limited understanding of the motivation for creative leisure pursuits in 'everyday life', and we cannot be completely sure about the role of creativity in preserving or promoting health and well-being. We know relatively little about why some older people take up creative leisure activities during retirement, widowhood or convalescence, while others do not. Such understanding could inform the design of health-promotion initiatives. A better understanding of the factors that encourage engagement in creative activities at different life stages would contribute to a better provision of creative opportunities within the community to boost psychological and social health. To better understand these issues we need further studies, especially those using self-report and phenomenological research methods, to reveal people's own 'insider' experience of the creative process. Such evidence would complement that gained from quantifying the creative outputs and career trajectories of eminent practitioners and the analysis of unusual case material by psychoanalytically trained researchers.

References

Albert R. Identity, experiences, and career choice among the exceptionally gifted and eminent. In: Runco M, Albert R (eds), Theories of Creativity. Newbury Park: Sage, 1990; 13–34.

Amabile T. Within you: without you: the social psychology of creativity, and beyond. In: Runco M, Albert R (eds). Theories of Creativity. Newbury Park: Sage, 1990; 61–91.

Bateson M. Composing a Life. New York, NY: Grove Press, 2001.

Becker G. The association of creativity and psychopathology: its cultural-historical roots. Creativity Research Journal 2000–2001; 13: 45–53.

Brown R. Creativity: what are we to measure? In: Glover J, Ronning R, Reynolds C (eds), Handbook of Creativity. New York, NY: Plenum, 1989; 3–32.

Chave A. O'Keeffe and the masculine gaze. Art in America 1990; 78: 114–24.

Christiansen C. Identity, personal projects and happiness: self construction in everyday action. Journal of Occupational Science 2000; 7: 98–107.

Cooper E. A critique of six measures for assessing creativity. Journal of Creative Behaviour 1991; 25, 194–204.

Csikszentmihalyi M. Flow: The Psychology of Optimal Experience. New York, NY: HarperCollins, 1990.

Day S. Make it uglier. Make it hurt. Make it real: narrative construction of the creative writer. Creativity Research Journal 2002; 14: 127–36.

Dekker K. Why oblique and why Jung? In: Pearson J (ed.), Discovering the Self through Drama and Movement. London: Jessica Kingsley, 1996; 39–45.

Domino G, Short J, Evans A, Romano P. Creativity and ego defence mechanisms: some exploratory empirical evidence. Creativity Research Journal 2002; 14: 17–25.

Dudek S, Croteau H. Aging and creativity in eminent architects. In: Adams-Price C (ed.), Creativity and Successful Aging: Theoretical and Empirical Approaches. New York, NY: Springer, 1998; 117–52.

Dudek S, Hall W. Personality consistency: eminent architects twenty-five years later. Creativity Research Journal 1991; 4: 213–31.

Fisher B, Specht D. Successful aging and creativity in later life. Journal of Aging Studies 1999; 13: 457–72.

Gedo J. More on creativity and its vicissitudes. In: Runco M, Albert R (eds), Theories of Creativity. Newbury Park: Sage, 1990; 35–45.

Gedo J. The Artist and the Emotional World: Creativity and Personality. New York, NY: Columbia University Press, 1996.

Gedo J. Psychoanalytic theories of creativity. In: Runco M (ed.), The Creativity Research Handbook (Vol. 1). Cresskill, NJ: Hampton Press, 1997; 29–39.

Helson R. Creativity in women: outer and inner views over time. In: Runco M, Albert R (eds), Theories of Creativity. Newbury Park, CA: Sage, 1990; 46–58.

Helson R. Ego identity and trajectories of productivity in women with creative potential. In: Adams-Price C (ed.), Creativity and Successful Aging: Theoretical and Empirical Approaches. New York, NY: Springer, 1998; 153–174.

Helson R. A longitudinal study of creative personality in women. Creativity Research Journal 1999; 12: 89–101.

Helson R, Pals J. Creative potential, creative achievement, and personal growth. Journal of Personality 2000; 68: 1–27.

Helson R, Roberts B, Agronick G. Enduringness and change in creative personality and the prediction of occupational creativity. Journal of Personality and Social Psychology 1995; 69: 1173–83.

Herrera H. Frida: A Biography of Frida Kahlo. London: Bloomsbury, 1998.

Jamison KF. Touched with Fire: Manic-depressive Illness and the Artistic Temperament. New York, NY: Simon & Schuster, 1993.

Kirschenbaum R, Reis S. Conflicts in creativity: talented female artists. Creativity Research Journal 1997; 10: 251–63.

Lehman H. Age and Achievement. Princeton, NJ: Princeton University Press, 1953.

Lindauer M. Artists, art, and arts activities: what do they tell us about aging? In: Adams-Price C (ed.), Creativity and Successful Aging: Theoretical and Empirical Approaches. New York, NY: Springer, 1998a; 237–50.

Lindauer M. Interdisciplinarity: the psychology of art and creativity: an introduction. Creativity Research Journal 1998b; 11: 1–10.

Lindauer M, Orwoll L, Kelley C. Aging artists on the creativity of their old age. Creativity Research Journal 1997; 10: 133–52.

Lubart T, Sternberg R. Life span creativity: an investment theory approach. In: Adams-Price C (ed.), Creativity and Successful Aging: Theoretical and Empirical Approaches. New York, NY: Springer, 1998; 21–41.

Marsiske M, Willis S. Practical creativity in older adults' everyday problem-solving: life span perspectives. In: Adams-Price C (ed.), Creativity and Successful Aging: Theoretical and Empirical Approaches. New York: Springer, 1998; 73–113.

Mishler E. Storylines: Craft Artists' Narratives of Identity. Cambridge, MA: Harvard University Press, 1999.

Orwoll L, Kelley M. Personal force and symbolic reach in older women artists. In: Adams-Price C (ed.), Creativity and Successful Aging. New York, NY: Springer, 1998; 175–94.

Reynolds F. Coping with chronic illness and disability through creative needlecraft. British Journal of Occupational Therapy 1997; 60: 352–6.

Reynolds F. Managing depression through needlecraft creative activities: a qualitative study. The Arts in Psychotherapy 2000; 27: 107–14.

Reynolds F. Reclaiming a positive identity in chronic illness through artistic occupation. OTJR: Occupation, Participation and Health 2003a; 23: 118–27.

Reynolds F. Conversations about creativity and chronic illness I: Textile artists coping with long-term health problems reflect on the origins of their interest in art. Creativity Research Journal 2003b; 15: 393–407.

Reynolds F, Prior S. 'A lifestyle coat-hanger': a phenomenological study of the meanings of artwork for women coping with chronic illness and disability. Disability and Rehabilitation 2003; 25: 785–94.

Richards R. Everyday creativity, eminent creativity and health: 'Afterview' for CRJ issues on creativity and health. Creativity Research Journal 1990; 3: 300–26.

Rodeheaver D, Emmons C, Powers K. Context and identity in women's late-life creativity. In: Adams-Price C (ed.), Creativity and Successful Aging. New York, NY: Springer, 1998; 195–234.

Schuldberg D. Schizotypal and hypomanic traits, creativity, and psychological health. Creativity Research Journal 1990; 3: 218–30.

Schwartz LL. Becoming a female artist: past, present and future. In: Bloom M, Gullotta T (eds), Promoting Creativity Across the Life Span. Washington, DC: CWLA Press, 2001; 191–230.

Simonton D. Age and literary creativity: a cross-cultural and transhistoric survey. Journal of Cross-Cultural Psychology 1975; 6: 259–77.

Simonton D. Age and outstanding achievement: what do we know after a century of research? Psychological Bulletin 1988; 104: 251–67.

Simonton D. Creativity in the later years: optimistic prospects for achievement. The Gerontologist 1990; 30: 626–31.

Simonton D. Career paths and creative lives: a theoretical perspective on late life potential. In: Adams-Price C (ed.), Creativity and Successful Aging: Theoretical and Empirical Approaches. New York: Springer, 1998; 3–18.

Simonton D. Creativity: cognitive, personal, developmental, and social aspects. American Psychologist 2000; 55: 151–8.

Simonton D. Underrepresented populations in creativity research. Creativity Research Journal 2002; 14: 279–80.

Slatkin W. The Voices of Women Artists. Englewood-Cliffs, NJ: Prentice-Hall, 1993.

Smith G, Lilja A, Salford L. Creativity and breast cancer. Creativity Research Journal 2002; 14: 157–62.

Tedeschi R, Calhoun L. Trauma and Transformation: Growing in the Aftermath of Suffering. New York, NY: Sage, 1995.

Zausner T. When walls become doorways: creativity, chaos theory and physical illness. Creativity Research Journal 1998; 11: 21–8.

CHAPTER 6

The effects of creativity on physical and psychological well-being: current and new directions for research

FRANCES REYNOLDS

Introduction

Having examined, in Chapter 5, some of the research into the influences that shape individual creativity, we now turn to studies that have explored the influence of creativity on physical and psychological well-being. This issue has not been much examined in mainstream creativity research. Simonton (2000) made this clear in his review of the state of research into creativity, when he described the principal objective of enquiry as being to explain the origins of human creativity, rather than to examine any of its psychological and social benefits.

Formulating valid research into the influence that creativity and creative occupation may have on well-being involves many difficulties. As noted previously, it seems that people who engage in creative occupations may already have certain psychological strengths, such as self-belief, tolerance for ambiguity, openness to experience and good levels of social support (Orwoll and Kelley, 1998). These resources may account for any positive health outcomes associated with creative engagement. Creative occupations also seem to increase the experience of control and choice (Reynolds and Prior, 2003). As perceived control is known to challenge depressed states of mind and to promote health, it is difficult to determine any additional ways in which creativity may promote well-being. In some forms of creative arts therapy, the artwork serves primarily as a means of forming a cohesive support group (for example, the cancer support group described by Heiney and Darr-Hope, 1999). In such cases, it is difficult to separate out the benefits attributable to the creative self-expression itself from those derived from the experience of support and commonality. People engage in a wide array of creative occupations, and the research literature is replete with investigations into different forms of visual art, creative writing, scientific discovery, entrepreneurial ventures and so on. Yet, the creativity inherent in many everyday forms of creativity (such as cooking, chess and other games, and team sports) has mostly been ignored. Our understanding of the health-promoting power of such activities is therefore minimal.

This chapter will focus broadly on the creative arts while acknowledging that there are many other types of creative occupation. It should be noted that findings about the health effects of the creative arts might not necessarily generalize to other forms of creativity. Four major types of research have increased our understanding of the influence of creativity upon health.

- Studies assessing the influence of creative occupations on lifestyle, health and well-being.
- Correlational studies in which health outcomes such as longevity are linked with participants' engagement in creative activities or to measures of their creativity.
- Observational accounts and interpretive analysis of the process and outcomes of art therapy sessions.
- Investigations that link physiological changes during creative activities to subsequent physical health outcomes.

We will see that research in this field is still at an early hypothesis-generating stage rather than providing any complete account of the effects of creativity upon health and well-being.

The influence of creative occupations on health and well-being

Many different research methods have been used to explore the influence of creativity and creative occupations on mental and physical health. Qualitative research allows access to personal experiences and the investigation of individuals' perceptions of the way in which creative occupation influences physical and psychological health. Phenomenological and grounded theory studies and questionnaire surveys have revealed how people perceive the effect of creative occupation on their well-being. For example, Clift and Hancox (2001) surveyed 84 members of a university choir to obtain their views on the health-promoting benefits of singing. They discovered that nearly everyone in the sample reported social benefits from being in the choir. Three-quarters of those sampled thought that they had gained emotional well-being and 58% thought that their physical health had improved. Many participants ascribed their better health to stress reduction and improved lung function. Although providing insights into possible health motives for participating in shared music-making, the study is limited by its focus on young people at university. Also, in common with many other questionnaire and interview studies, the research necessarily elicits participants' own perceptions of their enhanced health. More objective evidence of improvement in well-being following participation in the creative activity would, perhaps, be preferable.

Creativity and ageing

Some research has focused on the role of creativity in promoting successful ageing. For example, Fisher and Specht (1999) interviewed older people who were displaying their artwork at a local exhibition. Participants described their artwork as maintaining their involvement in the wider community, enabling personal growth and providing a productive focus to their lives, even in the face of physical limitations. Other evidence, for example Forthofer et al. (2001), shows self-esteem and social support networks to have positive influences on physical health and functioning so the health benefits of participating in community art projects warrant further research, as do the possible mechanisms linking creativity and health.

Some researchers have examined relationships between creativity and positive ageing through longitudinal studies. Vaillant and Vaillant (1990) examined some of the longitudinal data collected between 1921 and 1987 from an original sample of intellectually gifted children selected by Lewis Terman. Vaillant and Vaillant (1990) compared 20 of the most creative women remaining in the sample at 77 years of age with 20 of the least creative, to determine whether they differed in their satisfaction with life and adaptation to ageing. Even though the authors stated that they advocated a very general definition of creativity as 'putting something in the world that was not there before' (Vaillant and Vaillant, 1990, p. 607), they, in fact, assessed creativity in a way that gave prominence to public acclaim and creative careers. The system gave a score of one (the top mark) for state-wide recognition of a creative product, two for local community recognition for creativity (such as a published work), three for creative hobbies and four for little evidence of sustained creative activity.

In interview, at the age of 76–78 years, the women's adaptation to ageing was assessed on a five-point scale. Looking back at the data collected at previous assessment points in the women's lives, the researchers found that the highly creative individuals had been more satisfied with their work at 40 years old, and had been more active outside the home at 45 years old. They expressed more joy in living at 60 years old and were better adapted to ageing at 76–78 years of age. A similar association between creativity and positive attitudes towards ageing was found in an interview study of people aged 67–86 years (Smith and Van der Meer, 1990). Many of the highly creative women in the Vaillant and Vaillant (1990) study continued to be productive in their seventies, for example in writing, graphic art, musical recitals and sculpture. Vaillant and Vaillant (1990) also reported on certain other features of the women's lives, including the negative association between having a successful career and child-rearing, and the low mean lifetime income of the women compared with men in the study. They also found that having a highly supportive husband, or not having a husband at all, seemingly facilitated the careers of the highly creative group. Having a critical husband or bearing sole responsibility for parents tended to inhibit the women's creative development. However, the more and less creative individuals did not differ in their subjective appraisals of their own physical or mental health.

Caution must be exercised in interpreting these findings, as the research method cannot really establish definitively that a lifetime engagement in creative work enhances physical and mental health in old age. This is because the Terman study followed up a particularly advantaged sample of individuals, all of whom were recognized to be of very high intelligence at the outset. Only a small percentage was drawn from lower social class or ethnic minority families. Illustrating their privileged status, and contrary to the population at large, most of the Terman women went to excellent colleges in their youth despite the economic depression of the 1930s.

Also, we must acknowledge that the later analysis provided by Vaillant and Vaillant (1990) presents only one perspective on the women's creativity, because it gives precedence to public acclaim. Women who demonstrated everyday creativity, in home-making, for example, or who had numerous creative hobbies, scored low on their measurement scale. Their having 'low' creativity does not seem to be justified from the authors' description:

> *The twenty women categorized as less creative included many who had hobbies such as sewing, gardening, pottery glazing, or flower arranging; who were active in pastimes like dog shows, stamp collecting, or ornithology; or who, rather than being creative in, enjoyed taking courses in, art or folk dancing. However, their creative efforts were not known to have affected others outside their immediate and close friends.* (Vaillant and Vaillant, 1990; p. 612; authors' original italics)

It is open to debate whether people who take courses in art, or who seek to develop other creative skills, are less creative than those enjoying public acclaim. We might argue, from the work that associates openness to experience with creativity, that individuals who engage in life-long learning should also be regarded as creative (Wolfradt and Pretz, 2001). Nevertheless, taken overall, this longitudinal study is fascinating in revealing how social factors and role expectations can limit the flourishing of women's creativity, and how some women manage to achieve a late-life resurgence of their creative talents.

Creativity and chronic illness

Given its apparent contribution to the process of positive ageing, we might ask whether creativity promotes the health and well-being of people living with chronic illness and disability. Chronic illness affects much more than the physical body, and presents the person with numerous losses and stressful experiences, including loss of function, pain and changes to identity. Social stigma and barriers to normal community activities may also contribute to the illness experience. Furthermore, chronic illness often leads to loss of employment and other consequences, such as reduced standards of living and loss of social support networks (Hakim et al., 2000). Other usual activities also tend to be affected. For example, Wikström et al. (2001) found that people with rheumatoid arthritis reported a loss of about two-thirds of their leisure activities after the onset of their disease. As a result of all these losses, people often feel increasingly isolated, depressed, helpless and cut off from their familiar past self. Bury (1982) referred to these encompassing effects of illness using the term 'biographical disruption'. The stress of chronic illness may not only influence psychological well-being, but may have deleterious effects on the immune system, posing further risks to physical health (Evans et al., 2000).

Creative occupations appear to provide an effective antidote to many of the psychological difficulties presented by illness. Engagement in creativity seems to renew people's sense of agency and control, provides distraction from symptoms and illness anxieties, and sets meaningful goals. Reynolds (1997) collected written narratives from women who viewed their engagement in textile art as a means of living positively with chronic illness. Many of the women referred to their artwork as restoring a familiar and satisfactory self-image and relieving the negative feelings that were associated with illness, such as anxiety or depression. They described their creative activities as providing entry into new social networks, with the advantage that such relationships were based on mutual interests rather than illness. Almost all participants regarded creative pursuits as requiring deep concentration, enabling relaxation and helping to distract the mind from worries.

A subsequent study was based on in-depth interviews with 30 women living with chronic illness (Reynolds and Prior, 2003). Participants had a more extended opportunity to reflect on the contribution that their textile artwork made to their health and well-being. Artistic activities had many health-promoting functions. For example, they acted as a catalyst for many other satisfying activities, including social contact, travel and visits to exhibitions. They helped to fill the void that was left when illness forced retirement from work – enhancing vitality and motivation. Art was self-expressive and promoted personal growth and, for these reasons, helped some participants to feel, ultimately, that their illness had even been a blessing (Reynolds, 2003). Participants did not represent their artwork as solely promoting their psychological well-being. Some also considered that their physical health had benefited. For example, one participant said:

> I think it is ill-health or adverse things that make you look at creative things in a different light, they are absolutely essential. I think without it [textile artwork], it would have been harder to get back to the level of health that I've got to. (Reynolds and Prior, 2003, p. 792)

For people living with psychological difficulties, there is also some evidence that engagement in creative activities enhances well-being. For example, Perrins-Margalis et al. (2000) evaluated the effects of engaging in a six-week group programme of horticulture with 10 people with long-term mental health problems. The creative aspects of the activity were highly valued, with participants' life satisfaction, self-concept and well-being all improving, at least in the short term.

Further insights have been gained into people's broader creative strategies for managing life with chronic illness, beyond engagement in artistic pursuits. McWilliam et al. (1996) interviewed 13 older people (mean age 77 years) approximately five months and 12 months after a health-promotion intervention. This involved an opportunity, over a number of weeks, to engage in critical reflection about their lives, and their goals and strategies for enhancing their own lives and health, in the context of chronic illness. Participants recognized the active struggle in which they were engaged to overcome the effects of ill-health on everyday life. They emphasized the need to make the best use of their skills, and revealed their ingenuity for finding creative ways of gaining satisfaction, feelings of accomplishment, independence and quality of life. One participant said:

> Life is a wonderful thing, to enjoy every day, and see what you can accomplish . . . So, you can knit, or go outside and make a snowman. To me, you are doing something, rather than just sitting. (McWilliam et al., 1996, p. 4)

This study expands our understanding of creativity in everyday life by acknowledging that it encompasses more than artistic or imaginative leisure pursuits. Personally developed novel strategies may have a vital role to play in enhancing the quality of everyday life. The authors give an example of a woman who had discovered her own way of managing a colostomy bag, thereby gaining greater independence and self-esteem:

> The nurses didn't think I could maybe do it myself, and they were offering to come any time I needed it changed. And I said, 'No!' I have to conquer these things. So I put a mirror in my washbasin and there I stand. I had a long mirror, stood against the wall, but I couldn't seem to manipulate it the same. But I can, with this mirror in the washbasin. (McWilliam et al., 1996, p. 7)

This would not be considered as a 'creative' activity in most areas of creativity research, but clearly the participant had devised a novel solution to a pressing problem and had benefited accordingly. The researchers found that creativity was a central means of gaining quality of life in chronic illness, interpreting this widely to mean:

> new perspectives on purpose in life; new applications of personal, intergenerational, and spousal patterning; new solutions and alternatives to characteristic ways of doing and being; new understandings of themselves; and new expectations of life . . . All reflected the originality and meaningfulness characteristic of what is defined as 'everyday creativity'. (McWilliam et al., 1996, p. 13)

Much further research is needed into the subjective effects of creative strategies and occupations on well-being, particularly for those who are living with illness and impairment. Current qualitative research has shown that creativity is experienced as promoting health and well-being in diverse ways. Research has also found that people sometimes discover their creative interests and abilities *after* the onset of illness, suggesting that crisis can sometimes stimulate revision of priorities, lifestyle change and personal growth. However, research to date has been limited in focusing upon small, largely self-selected samples. Mostly women have been studied in the qualitative research which has been carried out to date, leaving uncertainty about men's perceptions of the health benefits of creative occupation.

What seems clear is that creativity is an aspect of meaningful occupation and promotes health. However, should we regard creativity as specifically health-promoting? Are other aspects of meaningful occupation equally or more important in promoting health? Other aspects of meaningful occupation include choice, social contact, intellectual stimulus and assertiveness. For example, other forms of occupation, including sporting activity and voluntary work, appear to increase the well-being of participants who live with chronic illness and impairment (Taylor and McGruger, 1996; Hainsworth and Barlow, 2001). Even quite simple interventions that give older people more decision-making power, choice, and responsibility within nursing homes, such as permission to alter furniture layout and caring for plants, have been shown to result in greater well-being, social interaction and alertness (Langer and Rodin, 1994). Although these aspects of meaningful occupation appear to be health-promoting, it appears that they have not necessarily been considered in association with creativity.

Research might focus on distinguishing the specific influences of creative strategies and creative activities on well-being, as opposed to interventions that generally enhance perceived control. Qualitative methods are valuable for providing access into participants' subjective worlds and for increasing our understanding of the personal significance of creative occupation. However, this approach to research cannot demonstrate, with any certainty, the causal influences involved, or determine whether and how creativity may restore physical functioning. The next section focuses on surveys that have attempted to estimate the effects of creative engagement upon physical health.

Linking physical health outcomes with creativity

Bygren et al. (1996) used a research design that overcame some of the limitations outlined above. They analysed data from a large interview survey of the living conditions, leisure activities and health of a random sample of Swedish people aged 16–74 years. Of particular focus for this study was the influence upon health of positive leisure activities, such as attending art exhibitions, concerts, cinema, theatre and sports events. The researchers also looked at the influence upon health of activities such as reading, making music and singing in a choir. They measured a number of factors that are known to influence health and mortality, such as age, sex, education level, income, presence of existing disease, social network, smoking habits and amount of physical exercise. These variables were statistically controlled in order to isolate and calculate the health-promoting influence of leisure activities.

Nearly 13,000 people were interviewed during 1982–3 and followed up again in 1991, when their survival was recorded. It was found that participants who reported more frequent attendance at cultural events at the start of the study were more likely to be still alive nine years later. When discussing their findings, the authors noted that confounding health-risk variables, such as disease and social network, were quite crudely measured, and therefore their precise effects on survival might not be judged with confidence. They also acknowledged that cultural attendance might reflect some other influential variable, such as personality, which could affect survival. Alcohol intake had not been assessed, and this too might be a confounding variable that influenced health and mortality.

While the researchers interpreted the data as confirming the health benefits of creative and other positive leisure activities, it remains uncertain whether people with fewer impairments and social stressors were better able to attend cultural events in the first place. Even with such complex statistical treatment, it is difficult to be certain about the direction of cause and effect.

Relatively few studies have attempted to evaluate the effects of creative activity on recovery from illness. One example was provided by Smith et al. (2002), who assessed creativity in women with breast cancer. This was done through the use of a laboratory-based test. This assessed participants' willingness to be flexible in interpreting a briefly presented visual image, through measuring the time taken to shift the initial interpretation. The researchers argued that the less perceptually fixed women were more open to their emotions, including aggression and anxiety. Openness to feelings, rather than suppression of them, seemed to be helpful in predicting a better outcome for certain types of breast cancer except the most aggressive, invasive type. Although the validity of the creativity measure used in this study must be debated, the method provides an intriguing example of a psychoanalytically guided, yet objective, enquiry into the relationship between creativity and physical health. It would be possible to extend such enquiry using a greater variety of measures of creative functioning.

Observing and interpreting creative art therapy

The creative therapies are usually regarded as comprising art, music, drama and dance movement therapies (Payne, 1993; Gilroy and Lee, 1995). Such forms of therapy offer clients the means to express themselves authentically, yet safely, in oblique, non-verbal ways (Dekker, 1996). The creative medium is seen as providing a container for raw emotions, and the therapeutic relationship provides further containment or holding. Adrian Hill (1951) discovered the value of art therapy in the 1930s during his stay, with tuberculosis, in a sanatorium. After many months, he took up drawing and painting and found that these activities gave him mental emancipation from the double confines of illness and hospitalization (Thomson, 1997).

Art therapists suggest that art-making is helpful for releasing and coming to terms with strong emotions, especially for clients with difficulties in verbal expression, such as people with learning difficulties, aphasia, clinical depression or enduring mental health problems. Art therapy may also have a healing effect on people who are wrestling with unspeakable emotions concerning life-threatening illness in children, adolescents or adults, or those who have suffered bereavement, trauma and abuse. Art therapists adopt various theoretical perspectives to guide their work, including Jung's psychodynamic approach and humanistic principles.

Art therapists have carried out relatively little formal research on the effectiveness of their work with clients. Edwards (1993) argued that lack of support and resources, as well as lack of training in research method-ologies, are potent barriers. A more recent survey of art therapists in the USA found similar reasons for their lack of involvement in research, including anxiety about statistics (Betts and Laloge, 2000). Restrictive, positivistic models of science may also deter art therapists, but qualitative methods, now more widely accepted, appear to offer acceptable and sub-tle ways of evaluating effectiveness, at least from the client's viewpoint.

Evaluations of art therapy outcomes are commonly based on the fol-lowing research strategies:

• therapists' interpretations of change in thematic expression during the course of therapy
• self-reports by clients
• objective changes in clients' behaviour.

A study by Fenton (2000) provides an example of a therapist interpreting clients' adjustment to cystic fibrosis through their changing styles of rep-resenting themselves in artwork. Children and adolescents may have a limited verbal capacity, and therefore art-making provides an effective, alternative means of communication about their feelings. Fenton argued that 'the language of the unconscious can speak where the conscious voice fails . . . Art making can promote feelings of self-esteem and improved body image, lessen feelings of isolation and synthesize spoken and unspoken fears' (Fenton, 2000, p. 17). She provided examples of the self-portraits drawn by three children with cystic fibrosis, interpreting possible meanings within each one. For example, one child drew a tree in the rain with clouds overhead. The therapist commented (Fenton, 2000, p. 22), 'Clouds are filled with moisture, as lungs are filled with mucus'. She also noted that the child, by leaving herself out of the picture, might be expressing 'feelings of isolation and separation' (Fenton, 2000, p. 22). Fenton argued that art could help children to process their unconscious fears and to develop new coping skills. Although the interpretations of the significance of the artwork appear open to debate, the health effects of creative self-expression could be evaluated through use of objective meas-ures. Fenton (2000) advocates further research into the medical changes that accompany art therapy.

Clients' experiences

A number of research studies, usually based on case material or qualitative interviews, have been carried out to explore clients' own experiences in art therapy. Predeger (1996) and Minar (1999) both examined the effects of creative art therapy on women with breast cancer. Minar (1999) did not offer a clear method but appeared to collect clients' own interpretations of their artwork as well as providing interpretations of her own. For example, one client created a self-portrait that she entitled 'Caught in a Whirlwind'. The client explained some of the themes within the picture: 'I felt like I was looking at my life from a distance, that it was someone else's life, not mine. I faced so many questions, decision and uncertainty – all swirling around! I had lost control' (Minar, 1999, p. 230).

Minar (1999, p. 230) interpreted the picture as representing 'the stabbing feeling, the fear of cancer'. She notes that, over time, the group members offered each other support, and that the women took from the creative process a renewed ability to cope with fear, and a new sense of purpose for their lives.

Predeger (1996) devised a co-operative or participatory research method in which women with breast cancer who took part in an art therapy group analysed for themselves the healing aspects of their art experiences. In common with the study above, Predeger (1996) suggested that the women's artwork expressed, directly or symbolically, the distress provoked by the illness and their disfiguring medical treatment. Creative artwork also helped the women to live positively with their illness by enabling them to focus more on the opportunities afforded by illness, rather than the losses that it had brought about. This change of perspective seemed likely to increase the women's resistance to depression. Some participants in Predeger's group commented on how their illness and confrontation with death had sharpened their perceptual awareness and appreciation of their lives and environment. The group had offered empowerment and reduced isolation. The creative process also offered escape from the illness experience through immersion in the colour and form of the artwork.

Piccirillo (1999) noted a similar effect among clients with HIV/AIDS who engaged in art. In certain respects, the art therapy experience seemed to confer certain psychological outcomes similar to those reported by the women who, as reviewed earlier, engaged in art as a leisure activity during chronic illness. However, art therapists are likely to be more attuned to unconscious meanings within the artwork than people engaging in art for leisure purposes. Even so, there is some evidence that lay artists appreciate some of the symbolic meanings within their work, at least in retrospect (Reynolds, 2002).

Objective measures of change in clients' health and functioning associated with art therapy

While most research into the effects of art therapy has drawn upon the perceptions of therapists and clients, some studies have attempted to monitor behavioural outcomes. Wigram (1993) assessed whether low-frequency sound in conjunction with music therapy could help calm people with learning difficulties and reduce their repetitive or self-injurious behaviour. An experimental design was used, with five clients allocated randomly to a music-only control condition and another five allocated to the experimental condition, where the music was accompanied by a pulsed, low-frequency tone. Behaviours such as rocking, picking at clothes and restless pacing were assessed before, during and after the sessions. No clear benefits emerged. It may be argued that the intervention did not involve creative responses on the part of the clients, although it was certainly designed to reduce non-creative, stereotypical behaviours. The research method is one that could be more widely attempted to gain objective data about changes in clients' functioning as a result of creative arts therapy.

Some comments on research into the effects of art therapy on health

Confident generalizations about the influence of creativity on well-being cannot be drawn from therapist and client reports of art therapy. This is because a particular type of person may elect to engage in this form of therapy; for example, a person who is comfortable with non-verbal expression and interested in the artistic medium offered.

Furthermore, therapeutic outcomes may not be only attributable to creative self-expression. The supportive relationship offered by the therapist provides a potentially powerful psychotherapeutic experience. Also, therapists' observations may be selective. Their own investment in the therapeutic process may lead to an overestimation of the positive outcomes of treatment. However, we need to recognize that bias can exist in other forms of research, too. To an outsider, some interpretations of the deeper meanings and effects of art-work appear open to dispute, as in the study by Fenton (2000). On the positive side, the combination of creative arts and psychotherapy training seems to equip art therapists with excellent skills for conceptualizing and assessing creativity and well-being, and for appreciating the unique benefits that creativity may bring to each client. Lindauer (1998) argued that research into creativity requires psychologists to have more understanding of art, just as art researchers require more understanding of psychology. His remark seems to apply to other disciplines, too. Art therapists seem to be in a good position to carry out such interdisciplinary research. Their sensitive, interpretive accounts of therapeutic processes and outcomes deepen our understanding of the possible health benefits of creative engagement and self-expression, and provide a number of hypotheses that could be tested in further, more systematic research.

It remains to be seen whether the arts therapies have demonstrable effects on physical health. Hiltebrand (1999) argued that art therapy might help people to externalize feelings that, if denied, might lead to physiological disturbance. Assessment of physiological change would offer another means of establishing the health-promoting power of creative art-making. This will be explored further in the next section.

Creativity and physical health outcomes: how are they linked?

In the last 15 years or so, research into the effects of stress on the functioning of the immune system has increased. This field is known as psycho-neuro-immunology. Much is now understood about the complexity of the immune system. It provides cell-mediated protection against viruses and cancer in the form of different types of white blood cell, known as lymphocytes, and also provides humoral-mediated protection in the form of antibodies. (*See* Evans et al., 2000, for details about the immune system and a review of research that examines how this system is affected by stress.) It has been shown that stress impacts on the immune system and therefore on health.

Psycho-neuro-immunology may hold the key to explaining why psychological factors such as low self-esteem and depression increase the risk of mortality, as shown by O'Connor and Vallerand (1998) in a prospective study of nursing home residents.

Creative arts activities seem to confer self-esteem and hope, and they enable self-expression that helps to alleviate stress and suppressed emotions. While the benefits of creativity may be understood in purely psychological terms, it would be valuable to know whether creative engagement promotes physical health directly through restoring healthy immune function.

Pennebaker and colleagues (1988) conducted the main body of research in this area, using experimental methods to examine the ways in which writing about traumatic experiences affects immune function, compared with writing about neutral topics. In most of their studies, short essays are written in private, usually on four consecutive days. Undergraduates have shown improved immune function in precursors of T-lymphocytes and reduced visits to a health centre in the six weeks following the intervention (Pennebaker et al., 1988). Pennebaker and colleagues interpreted the findings by suggesting that the suppression of memories and feelings about a traumatic experience created long term stress, and that writing privately about such experiences can alleviate such stress, with beneficial effects on immune functioning (Petrie et al., 1998). They also argued that non-verbal expression, through art, music and other therapies, may possibly have an impact on health, particularly if accompanied by verbal processing (Berry and Pennebaker, 1993).

Research into the health-promoting consequences of creative engagement upon the immune system has hardly begun. The research into writing about emotional experiences is somewhat limited by its almost exclusive focus upon undergraduates and neglect of other groups within the population. Student samples tend to be socially advantaged, and, by virtue of their youth, not all of those participating have encountered profoundly distressing life events. It is unclear whether people who are disturbed by serious physical or mental health problems would necessarily show the same benefits from engaging in very brief episodes of personal writing.

The immune system is highly complex and responds differently to short-term and long-term stressors. Participants in the personal writing studies have tended to be followed up for only short periods, making it difficult to ascertain with confidence any longer term health benefits. Nevertheless, studies into the effects on immune functioning of engaging in creative activities are urgently needed. Relatively non-invasive procedures are available, such as measuring the levels of cortisol or secretory immunoglobulin A in saliva, and these allow comparative measures to be taken before and after individuals engage in creative tasks. It may be possible, also, to correlate subjective self-reports, such as relief from depression or increase in self-esteem, with the measurements taken of immune functioning.

Some of the other measures used in psycho-neuro-immunology research, such as vulnerability to respiratory infection or speed of recovery from surgery, may also provide means of establishing whether individuals who engage more extensively in creative activities have objectively better physical health outcomes. Nevertheless, complex research designs will be needed to disentangle the specific health benefits of creative activity from other potential therapeutic experiences associated with such activities, such as increased personal control or social support.

New directions for research

Assessing psychological and physical outcomes

The review above has shown that numerous research methods have been used to explore the influence of creativity and creative occupation on health. Several critiques of existing research have been presented, and certain modifications and extensions to this research have been suggested. Qualitative methods have been very useful for giving fresh insights into the contribution that creative occupation makes to psychosocial well-being, but such methods do not lend themselves to establishing whether and how creativity may result in measurable improvements to physical health. Surveys, although limited in number, suggest that creative involvement may confer health benefits, at least in the realms of social and psychological functioning. However, such methods cannot generally disentangle cause and effect, making it difficult to be sure that creativity is really promoting good health, rather than simply reflecting participants' pre-existing levels of well-being. The accounts of art therapists offer many hypotheses about the therapeutic impact of creativity that is expressed within the confines of a safe therapeutic context. Larger scale research could be useful to establish whether some of the findings are replicable and to evaluate the impact of creative therapies upon physical health, as this has been hardly investigated at all. As discussed above, studies that have examined stress physiology, using non-invasive procedures such as testing salivary cortisol, hold much promise for linking physiological and psychological aspects of health. Such methods would complement qualitative enquiry into the subjective meaning of creative occupation by establishing whether satisfying, self-expressive activities diminish the physiological stress response. In the context of chronic illness, it may also be possible to compare the disease activity, functional performance and other health indicators of groups of people who do and do not engage regularly in creative leisure pursuits.

Gender differences

Although traditional creativity research, which concentrated on the origins of creativity, focused largely on men, a number of recent studies have sought to understand how women discover and express their creativity. This has resulted in a number of studies of female artists and other eminent creative women. Many report discovering their creative interests and talents in mid-life and later years, suggesting that research might examine in more detail this process of discovery. Better understanding of the personal, social and cultural supports for creativity might help to suggest how to set up attractive opportunities for creativity in middle and later life. This could assist in the effective promotion of public health.

Whilst there have been many studies of eminent creative men, it is unclear whether and how men, in the general population, express their creative potential, and what psychological, social and health benefits they may derive. Masculine identities tend to be grounded in attributes such as physical strength and activity. Cultural notions of hegemonic masculinity inhibit men's emotional self-awareness and self-expression, and this inhibition may limit men's interests in the creative arts. Because we are still limited in our understanding and definitions of creativity, we clearly need more qualitative enquiry into men's general understanding of its meaning and relevance to their everyday lives and health.

Likewise, the psychological benefits that some women describe from participating in the creative arts need further investigation. Some research suggests that the social and cultural context is an important enabling factor promoting women's engagement in creative activities. It may be possible to further disentangle the relative importance of social support and creative activity in promoting health. If creative pursuits lead to an expansion of social support networks, then these creative activities may be expected to have valuable health-promoting consequences in their own right. Research is needed with larger, random samples (for example, of older adults joining creative arts adult education classes) to examine inter-relationships between creative occupation, social support networks and ensuing health.

Randomized controlled trials

The randomized controlled trial is usually held to be the pre-eminent research method in clinical and health research for demonstrating the health benefits of an intervention. It would be intriguing to randomly allocate people with chronic illness to a new creative leisure activity or a non-creative leisure activity (if definitions of what should be counted as creative can be agreed). Similar research designs (for example, Lamb et al., 2002) have been used to investigate the health-promoting effects of physical exercise. Assessments could be made over time of any physical, social and psychological health benefits that accrue specifically to involvement in a creative leisure activity compared with a control group.

Although this research design would provide a powerful tool for estimating the extent to which creative occupation is accessible, satisfying and health-promoting for clients with ill-health, we must recognize that there are numerous barriers to conducting such a trial. Given individual differences in personality, interests, skills, family background and professional identity – all of which are likely to affect choice of preferred creative activity – it would be unwise to allocate patients randomly to a single creative or control activity. A creative activity that appeals to one person may seem uninteresting, anxiety-provoking or patronizing to another. Also, unless restrained within a hospital setting, the control patients might well engage in other forms of meaningful creative activity as part of their daily lifestyle at home, such as gardening or creative cookery. Although randomized controlled trials are a preferred means of evaluating therapy, their use to control people's leisure activities in the community may be considered unethical. However, a quasi-experimental field design might be feasible, as has been used in other health promotion initiatives such as the Stanford Five-City Heart Project, in which opportunities for physical activity, health education and health counselling were introduced into some communities and not into others (Farquhar et al., 1985). Over time, participation rates in various health-promoting activities, health knowledge and ensuing cardiac health outcomes in the different communities were compared. Similarly designed initiatives could result in the comparison of health outcomes in communities that provide an increased number of creative opportunities, against those that maintain the status quo.

Defining creative occupation

As discussed in the previous chapter, research into the health-promoting power of creative occupation has been made difficult by limited and contested definitions of creativity. Reis (2001) argued that women, in particular, diversify their creative interests into home tasks (such as decorating, budgeting, scheduling and multi-tasking), nurturing relationships, service to others and personal appearance, as well as engaging in conventionally defined creative work and hobbies. If creativity is seen as optimal functioning (Runco, 2001), or as a 'resolution of a challenge involving unknowns, whose solution has social value' (Bloom and Gullotta, 2001, p. 7) then perhaps we need to include a much wider array of everyday activities under the umbrella of creativity. Games and sports that involve complex problem-solving to gain a result that is unpredictable at the outset may also be considered as creative. The inclusion of such occupations helps to prevent an overly narrow focus upon the health-promoting possibilities of the creative arts. Furthermore, Cropley (1990) argued that mental health may be promoted by helping people to attack everyday situations with creative strategies, rather than through training programmes designed to increase abstract creativity or the abilities valued by creativity tests. This form of mental health promotion holds much promise but continues to be neglected.

Conclusion

This chapter has introduced a wide range of research exploring the complex inter-relationships that occur between creativity and health. While
many participants, particularly in the creative arts, report psychological and
physical health benefits, more research is needed to determine whether
objective changes in functioning can be detected and to elucidate the critical processes involved. From this overview, it can be argued that definitions
of creativity need to be revisited, more everyday forms of creativity need to
be acknowledged and studied, and more evidence is required about the
physiological mechanisms through which creative activities may exert influence over physical health. Nevertheless, the research to date offers a
positive view of people's capacity to discover their creativity in later life, and
to embark on creative activities which promote mental well-being and, perhaps, physical health, even in the context of chronic illness and other
adversities. The field seems ripe for vigorous further enquiry.

References

Berry D, Pennebaker J. Nonverbal and verbal emotional expression and health.
Psychotherapy and Psychosomatics 1993; 59: 11–19.

Betts D, Laloge L. Art therapists and research: a survey conducted by the Potomac
Art Therapy Association. Art Therapy 2000; 17: 291–5.

Bloom M, Gullotta T. Creativity and primary prevention: terms of engagement. In:
Bloom M, Gullotta T (eds), Promoting Creativity across the Life Span.
Washington, DC: CWLA Press, 2001; 1–16.

Bury M. Chronic illness as biographical disruption. Sociology of Health and
Illness 1982; 4: 167–82.

Bygren L, Konlaan B, Johansson S. Attendance at cultural events, reading books
or periodicals, and making music or singing in a choir as determinants of survival: Swedish interview survey of living conditions. British Medical Journal
1996; 313: 1577–80.

Clift S, Hancox G. The perceived benefits of singing: findings from preliminary
surveys of a university college choral society. Journal of the Royal Society for
the Promotion of Health 2001; 121: 248–56.

Cropley A. Creativity and mental health in everyday life. Creativity Research
Journal 1990; 3: 167–78.

Dekker K. Why oblique and why Jung? In: Pearson J (ed.), Discovering the Self
through Drama and Movement. London: Jessica Kingsley, 1996; 39–45.

Edwards D. Why don't arts therapists do research? In: Payne H (ed.), Handbook
of Inquiry in the Arts Therapies: One River, Many Currents. London: Jessica
Kingsley, 1993; 7–15.

Evans P, Hucklebridge F, Clow A. Mind, Immunity and Health: The Science of
Psychoneuroimmunology. London: Free Association Books, 2000.

Farquhar J, Fortmann S, Maccoby N, Haskell W, Williams P, Flora J et al. The Stanford Five-City Project: design and methods. American Journal of Epidemiology 1985; 122: 323–34.

Fenton JF. Cystic fibrosis and art therapy. The Arts in Psychotherapy 2000; 27: 15–25.

Fisher B, Specht D. Successful aging and creativity in later life. Journal of Aging Studies 1999; 13: 457–72.

Forthofer M, Janz N, Dodge J, Clark N. Gender differences in the associations self esteem, stress and social support with functional health status among older adults with heart disease. Journal of Women and Aging 2001; 13: 19–36.

Gilroy A, Lee C (eds). Art and Music: Therapy and Research. London: Routledge, 1995.

Hainsworth J, Barlow J. Volunteers' experiences of becoming arthritis self-management lay leaders: 'It's almost as if I've stopped aging and started to get younger!' Arthritis and Rheumatism 2001; 45: 378–83.

Hakim E, Bakheit A, Bryant T, Roberts M, McIntosh-Michaelis S, Spackman A et al. The social impact of multiple sclerosis: a study of 305 patients and their relatives. Disability and Rehabilitation 2000; 22: 288–93.

Heiney S, Darr-Hope H. Healing Icons: art support program for patients with cancer. Cancer Practice 1999; 7: 183–9.

Hill A. Painting Out Illness. London: Williams & Norgate, 1951.

Hiltebrand E. Coping with cancer through image manipulation. In: Malchiodi C (ed.), Medical Art Therapy with Adults. London: Jessica Kingsley, 1999; 113–36.

Lamb S, Bartlett H, Ashley A, Bird W. Can lay-led walking programmes increase physical activity in middle-aged adults? A randomised controlled trial. Journal of Epidemiology and Community Health 2002; 56: 246–52.

Langer E, Rodin J. The effects of choice and enhanced personal responsibility for the aged: a field experiment in an institutional setting. In: Steptoe A, Wardle J (eds), Psychosocial Processes and Health: A Reader. Cambridge: Cambridge University Press, 1994; 400–12.

Lindauer M. Interdisciplinarity: the psychology of art and creativity: an introduction. Creativity Research Journal 1998; 11: 1–10.

McWilliam C, Stewart M, Brown J, Desai K, Coderre P. Creating health with chronic illness. Advances in Nursing Science 1996; 18: 1–15.

Minar V. Art therapy and cancer: images of the hurter and healer. In: Malchiodi C (ed.), Medical Art Therapy with Adults. London: Jessica Kingsley, 1999; 227–42.

O'Connor B, Vallerand R. Psychological adjustment variables as predictors of mortality among nursing home residents. Psychology of Aging 1998; 13: 368–74.

Orwoll L, Kelley M. Personal force and symbolic reach in older women artists. In: Adams-Price C (ed.), Creativity and Successful Aging. New York, NY: Springer, 1998; 175–94.

Payne H. (ed.), Handbook of Inquiry in the Arts Therapies: One River, Many Currents. London: Jessica Kingsley, 1993.

Pennebaker J, Kiecolt-Glaser J, Glaser R. Disclosure of traumas and immune function: health implications for psychotherapy. Journal of Consulting and Clinical Psychology 1988; 56: 239–45.

Perrins-Margalis N, Rugletic J, Schepis N, Stepanski H, Walsh M. The immediate effects of a group-based horticulture experience on the quality of life of persons with chronic mental illness. Occupational Therapy in Mental Health 2000; 16: 15–32.

Petrie K, Booth R, Pennebaker J. The immunological effects of thought suppression. Journal of Personality and Social Psychology 1998; 75: 1264–72.

Piccirillo E. Beyond words: the art of living with AIDS. In: Malchiodi C (ed.), Medical Art Therapy with Adults. London: Jessica Kingsley, 1999; 163–88.

Predeger E. Womanspirit: a journey into healing through art in breast cancer. Advances in Nursing Science 1996; 18: 48–58.

Reis S. Toward a theory of creativity in diverse creative women. In: Bloom M, Gullotta T (eds), Promoting Creativity across the Life Span. Washington, DC: CWLA Press, 2001; 231–76.

Reynolds F. Coping with chronic illness and disability through creative needlecraft. British Journal of Occupational Therapy 1997; 60: 352–6.

Reynolds F. Symbolic aspects of coping with chronic illness through textile arts. The Arts in Psychotherapy 2002; 29: 99–106.

Reynolds F. Reclaiming a positive identity in chronic illness through artistic occupation. OTJR: Occupation, Participation and Health 2003; 23: 118–27.

Reynolds F, Prior S. 'A lifestyle coat-hanger': a phenomenological study of the meanings of artwork for women coping with chronic illness and disability. Disability and Rehabilitation 2003; 25: 785–94.

Runco M. Creativity as optimal human functioning. In: Bloom M, Gullotta T (eds). Promoting Creativity across the Life Span. Washington DC: CWLA Press, 2001; 17–44.

Simonton D. Creativity: cognitive, personal, developmental, and social aspects. American Psychologist 2000; 55: 151–8.

Smith G, Van der Meer G. Creativity in old age. Creativity Research Journal 1990; 3: 249–64.

Smith G, Lilja A, Salford L. Creativity and breast cancer. Creativity Research Journal 2002; 14: 157–62.

Taylor L, McGruger J. The meaning of sea kayaking for persons with spinal cord injuries. American Journal of Occupational Therapy 1996; 50: 39–46.

Thomson M. On Art and Therapy: An Exploration. London: Free Association Books, 1997.

Vaillant G, Vaillant C. Determinants and consequences of creativity in a cohort of gifted women. Psychology of Women Quarterly 1990; 14: 607–16.

Wigram T. The feeling of sound: the effect of music and low frequency sound in reducing anxiety and challenging behaviour in clients with learning difficulties. In: Payne H (ed.), Handbook of Inquiry in the Arts Therapies: One River, Many Currents. London: Jessica Kingsley, 1993; 177–96.

Wikström I, Isacsson Å, Jacobsson T. Leisure activities in rheumatoid arthritis: change after disease onset and associated factors. British Journal of Occupational Therapy 2001; 64: 87–92.

Wolfradt U, Pretz J. Individual differences in creativity: personality, story writing and hobbies. European Journal of Personality 2001; 15: 297–310.

CHAPTER 7

Individual accounts of the effect of creative activity on health and well-being

COMPILED AND EDITED BY THERESE SCHMID

'The best things in life are free'

> Words and music by BG DeSylva, Lew Brown and
> Ray Henderson, 1927; recorded by Dinah Shore, 1948.

Introduction

What useful purpose would be served by writing this book if it did not talk of how people feel about their experiences with creativity? I could tell many of my own, but I have found that when I have discussed the argument of the book, with many people, in many situations, the responses have always been to the effect that it should be obvious to everyone that the creativity we all have is one of our greatest assets, and should be highly valued and understood.

The following contributions were gathered from people who were interested in writing about the effects of creative activities on their health and well-being. Some of the contributors have an illness or have recovered from an illness, and for them creativity has been a blessing. For others it has been one of the pleasures of life. Many other people will tell the same story. This chapter provides a glimpse into the positive effects on well-being that creativity offers people who have an illness and those who are not ill. This is the argument of the book. The accounts speak for themselves and no conclusions will be drawn. It is not intended to represent a research project; however, like Chapter 9, it is assumed that useful consensual truth can be derived from the collection, that may suggest opportunities for research.

A written invitation and information letter was sent to people who were known to me or who were suggested to me, and they were asked to write a brief account of their experiences with creativity. They were asked whether their experiences gave them feelings such as pleasure, joy, excitement, confidence, satisfaction, self-esteem, feeling connected and a sense of belonging and, if so, whether those feelings contributed to their health and well-being.

All the responses received have been included, and nearly all of the requests for accounts received a response. Many of the accounts have been prepared by people with limited or no experience in writing about such experiences, but all were happy to try. Interestingly, all of the accounts are from women.

Two accounts are from performers of the Performing Older Women's Circus, Vig Geddes and Saralyn, who I met whilst they were on tour in Albury and Wodonga, NSW, Australia, in 2003. The ages of members range from 40 to 71 years. I met Rita Sheahan, in Gundagai, NSW, in 2002. Rita had just published a book, that was the fulfilment, in her later life, of a dream. Mary Ewington was suggested by a friend. Katrina Varian was suggested by editor and lecturer Rosemary Caultron, New Zealand. I met Marley Critcher at the local Spinners and Weavers Guild, and became aware of her skills with music, knitting and spinning. Rita Wenberg, an Aboriginal artist, I met through a contact made with an Aboriginal Community Development officer at a local council. I met Eve Gray at a Spinners and Weavers Guild, having been inspired by her short story, 'Merino', in *Songs of the Unsung Heroes. Stories and Verse Celebrating Australian Women and Their Work* (Australian Workers Heritage Centre, 2002, Queensland, Australia). Siobhan heard about my interest in this subject from Paul Brewer, the co-ordinator of Sound Minds, Battersea, London.

All contributors are active in doing creative activities in their lives and were motivated to do so for various reasons. The accounts include descriptions of creativity in the assistance of a recovery from an illness or as assistance during the process of enduring an illness. Most accounts illustrate that creativity is lived as a way of life. The contributions are open for interpretation in all sorts of ways, for example: in examining motivation; in considering the semantics of the word *creativity*; in examining creativity as an attitude, a way of life that is filtered through all everyday activities; and in investigating creative activities as a diversion from the negative, psychological impact of an illness, disability or dysfunction, to name a few.

The nine contributions are:

- 'Creativity and expression *is* the real thing'.
- 'Getting out there – *Barney the White Cockatoo*'.
- 'A place of integration'.
- 'Finding ways to show off'.
- 'Expanding horizons'.
- 'Fun, challenges and endless surprises'.
- 'Thank goodness for my painting'.
- 'A feeling of wholeness'.
- 'Creativity comes from love'.

Creativity and expression *is* the real thing

Mary Hudson Ewington, Mount Nelson, Tasmania, Australia

Mary Hudson Ewington has a CD-ROM: 'Seasons of Fruitfulness', on which she compiled images and text whilst she was undergoing treatment for breast cancer. She performs with the 'Deep Listening' a cappella group and composes songs, *Southern Stars*. Mary produces a magazine of her students' writing, *Versions Magazine*, and has published three editions of the anthology *Versions Writing and Graphics* (1987, 1992, 1994). She has completed her masters degree in Educational Studies (2003) and Certificate in Initiatic Art Therapy (2004).

The first story I have to write comes from my deepest being – and somewhere else. My art is important. I have written, painted and sung most of my life, and used it for my enjoyment. I keep finding I am so fortunate. My images (paintings, cartoons and drawings) and writing (journal, short stories, poetry and songs) got me through my chemotherapy and continue to give me a sense of myself. Making art and writing is a way of externalizing internal impulses, so saving wear and tear on the body and mind. In fact they connect me with the greater intelligence, emotion, physicality and spirituality. Directly.

How odd, out of this world and weird it was, being drugged. I do remember a time when I explored another world, a world deeper and other than anything I have known before.

I had reacted strongly to the first chemotherapy, getting dehydrated, nauseous and anxious. Lorazepam did not help sufficiently. I went to Emergency and then to hospital where I stayed five days. (There, I wrote a murder mystery, drew terrifying pictures and cried to the social worker.) After this scary time my doctor and I decided I should book myself into hospital for the second treatment, so my sister and I waited for the nurse to hook my arm to the chemicals without spilling a dangerous drop on my bare skin. I then lay down and submitted. (I drew pictures of my poor hand, with various drips.)

Gradually I felt worse. I vomited with monotonous regularity. The staff were solicitous and gave me a stomach drip and an anti-nausea drug. I had to sit it out and hope it would eventually ease up. I had an intense headache. My legs started twitching. I ate ice and sipped water – 12 cups per day to flush the drugs through. All thoughts of anything but my body fled the room. I could do nothing but moan and cry. I later drew a cartoon of me as a baby, asking my Dad/my partner to pick me up and carry me out of there: 'Please. Literally, take me!'.

Lorraine phoned the next afternoon, 'Can I come and give you Light?' 'Sure, about half an hour.' She sat by me and opened her palms near my kidneys, head and breast areas. I moaned. I ached. I could not escape this black depth of what seemed my imminent death. There was nowhere to go. I breathed. I focused. I tried to relax. I twitched. My legs jumped. I tried to lie still. Forget about it. All to no avail. Lorraine's presence was soothing. She stayed. I eventually gave up. This death would last forever. Who cared? Not me.

Suddenly I found under the blackness a space. Not light and sweet, but a space, a new space. Below the aching body, below and away from depression, away from whatever death could be. It was solace. I opened up to a new space of me. It has proven to be my strength and has never left me. This space connects me to my inner self, my self-value, my right to my life, my choices. It has made me less tolerant of whingeing, whining and complaining, and gives me the strength to cut through others' crap and excuses. It has also made me more compassionate of others' hardships. Artwork and writing every day expresses me, well, happy, sick or isolated. At times I become so excited at what I can find, I become high on art. I express visually what I cannot write and vice versa. Among the illness I recovered my power and regained a sense of wellness, humour, intrigue and fun. I don't want to forget the bare bones, and I can't forget the blackness. It is me.

The second story follows from my being a client or patient. While I was ill, my a cappella group 'Deep Listening' came to sing to me. I learnt singing is great lying down, as I was so used to running the group, standing up and working hard. I was honoured that they visited and gave me a concert. What a gift. The actual sounds soothed, roused, elevated my mood, caused me to sit up and play the guitar! I experienced feelings of pleasure, confidence, satisfaction, self-esteem and an improvement in health and well-being (mental, emotional, spiritual, physical and social), arising from these feelings.

I talked about these activities with my hospital psychologist. She mentioned how well I was coping after the initial shock of diagnosis and treatment. In contrast, so many women are isolated and struggle, having little income, children, and often their partner leaves. I would visit her with a new song, pictures or a story, even though some were very black. She said she looked forward to my appointments and reassured me I was completely sane.

Mentally, I composed new songs – 'Chemotherapy' and 'Scoparia' for the Thanksgiving Concert; emotionally, I felt a sense of receiving; spiritually, the songs we sing are uplifting and designed to be so; physically, I relaxed and had some fun; socially, I enjoyed my friends' attention and voices. I felt well after each visit. It was a real physical change. The group has met each week since 1996, and after two hours of singing and heavy breathing we feel like going out and dancing all night. Our energy rises, we feel connected, powerful, and it shows so obviously when we meet others. You can immediately tell who is 'not present'.

There is deep personal growth in expression, a family connection according to Virginia Satir, and social meaning and connection, shown in many festivals. For example, the Wake of a Buddhist friend was beautifully sung and drummed with deep spiritual feeling by about 50 people. It showed me that we have taken 10 years, with celebrations, kirtans, meditation, workshops, exhibitions and time at the beach, to learn the songs, harmonize, find spiritual comfort with each other, celebrate death, beauty, wilderness and share food by the fireside.

I have used art, writing and music all my life. I have always known their benefits for me in my creativity, mood, attention for others, teaching situations and for the community. However, I always thought of them as being icing on the cake of work. I now know that creativity and expression *is* the work, the essence, the real thing. For example, when kids in a classroom mucked about and drew doodles, or coloured in patterns and threaded beads, I had thought they were wasting 'thinking' time. I now know that they are benefiting by this real activity as part of their present reality, not even as some preparation for the future, and that non-thinking and feeling is deeper and more connecting than thinking. It is not a comparison but a different space. They can have a sense of acceptance in the art or drama room, depending on the awareness of the teacher.

I teach art therapy privately, intentionally for healing and for wellness. For years I taught re-evaluation counselling and saw creativity as a high level of expression, different from emotional neediness or 'clienting', 'tho some artists express neediness in their art' (Juan Davilla). Singing is a wellness activity, as you can't cry and sing at the same time. I teach creative writing and recognize that we create stories that serve to make sense of the world, including for therapeutic value. This doesn't mean that we must be sick to start with. There is a continuum from sickness to wellness, and arts can be used at all stages and for all purposes, the more the better.

Getting out there – *Barney the White Cockatoo*

Rita Sheahan, Gundagai, NSW, Australia

Writing my story was a great way of getting out there and allowing my imagination to run free, it was also the realization of a kind of dream. I always wanted to do it, and at 73 years old I felt time was running away. It was like now or never!

I have always believed in the words of the old song, 'The Best Things in Life are Free'. My story was written mainly as a 'keepsake from grandma', for my many grandchildren. I wished to remind them to appreciate the wonderful, mysterious and beautiful gifts of nature that surround us, and are so often taken for granted. And also, to enjoy the unique animal, bird life and flora we have in our great country.

The white cockatoo was chosen as the central character because he is intelligent and garrulous. Although the story is set in a time of drought, there was still space to remark on the purple hills in spring, the radiant dawn and the glowing sunsets. The story tells how a farming family existed through tough times as well as good times with courage and good faith.

I thoroughly enjoyed completing this long-delayed project. Although I published a few copies myself, at some expense, the response of the people who have read *Barney the White Cockatoo* is very pleasing. Apart from the editor and illustrators, who all gave me good support, it was not a group project. I have gained much pleasure and a sense of achievement that I was able to publish my story.

A place of integration

Vig Geddes, Performing Older Women's Circus, Victoria, Australia

One of the things that I notice about physical performance is that it is one of the few places in my life where I feel totally whole, where all aspects of my being are working as one. A place where my imagination, my intelligence and my physical body are all integrated. Sometimes I feel like there is also spiritual dimension in acrobalance, when Bridget and I are working together, very focused on one another, and when our breathing is in sync. It feels like we are one with each other, with Kim's music, with the show and with the audience, and that is deeply satisfying.

The best I ever feel about myself is when we are intensively rehearsing a show, or when we are doing a season. I think it is partly the physical fitness – that is the time when I am at my fittest – and partly it is because of all the things I have described above. When that is happening I feel free and fluid, and able to be whoever I want to be. I feel very outgoing and positive about the world and myself. For me, there is something exciting and satisfying about being very 'in my body' while at the same time trying to convey emotions, images and stories.

We have a lot of fun together in the Performing Older Women's Circus (POW), and, because the core business of what we are doing together is performance, the fun tends to be around performance activities, like playing music or singing together, doing imitations of each other, of people we meet, of koalas or cockatoos, making up little ditties about each other, making up stories, retelling and embellishing stories, making up jokes, just being silly. The culture of POW supports and encourages creativity of any kind. So, when we are together at rehearsals or shows, it feels to me like we have permission to be or do anything so long as it is not going to be hurtful to any one. In fact, we encourage each other to do this. In this setting, POW women often try things, both on- and off-stage, that they might not have done outside POW. For me, the anticipation before a POW season is about fun, creativity, being allowed and encouraged to go over the top and have some very dynamic interactions with other women.

Although I have some interesting and entertaining friends, with whom I have fun, there is something about the performance and physical training with others that provides something else that makes a total 'mind and body' experience. I imagine that people who do ballroom dancing might say something similar.

Finding ways to show off

Saralyn, Performing Older Women's Circus, Victoria, Australia

I have been part of the Performing Older Women's Circus (POW) for almost two years, and it is good not to feel new. At the same time I still feel like a toddler compared with some of the women whose skills are so much more developed than mine. It's exciting to know all that there is ahead of me to learn. The skills I have learnt are to be a base for various acrobalances, such as bluebird, car seat, candlestick, foot sit. I can hold up other women with my feet and hands, and it is an achievement to be able to use any of these balances in a show. The trainers respect the physical limits we have, but also encourage and challenge us to push out those limits by trying new things. I have developed more self-confidence to be able to perform but also to walk more confidently through life. Again, I look forward to increasing skills in that area.

I find the process of creating a new show a fascinating one. It is filled with creativity from start to finish. We have input into the written material which is collected to make the script. This is creative, as stories are written, then acted out. We also have some say in shaping various images with our bodies, coming up with ideas for how to be the props, for example furniture or landscape. The director starts us off with enthusiasm and then leaves it up to us to work things out. Working in small groups, the ideas seem to generate from each other and some are discarded and others kept. The ideas don't have someone's name on them: they are group property. There is a place for everyone's skill level. For example, when forming a garden, those who can do a balance to make an archway do that, and someone else might be a flower or a fountain. We usually have to think quickly to come up with the ideas and then present them to the rest of the group, and this is also good as spontaneity is not a strong point for me.

Two things happened around the same time and I don't remember which came first to influence me joining the POW. I was seeing a counsellor about an issue around a loss in my life. She challenged me to take more risks, to find ways to show off and to bring my inner and outer life closer together. She knew of POW and encouraged me to enquire as a challenge. The other personal encounter was through a friend who must have known that the POW would be just the thing for me, because one day over coffee, she presented it to me in glowing terms. She is a 'Women's Circus' member, but knew of POW and saw how much fun it was for those involved. I took the leap and joined without knowing anyone, and found myself in a supportive and friendly group that affirmed my attempts. I thought weekly Saturday afternoon training times were quite a commitment and I didn't even know about show rehearsals! But now, I don't know what else I'd rather do during that time. My family doesn't complain about my absence because they know I'm doing something that makes me happy. Friends and family support me by coming to the shows and it's great to have them proud of what I do.

I know that participation has increased my health and well-being. I still have low energy at times in spite of the increased exercise (including gym workouts twice a week) but it isn't as frequent. Chronic pain, partially due to arthritis, has lessened as well. Even when it is there, it is better to be doing something fun and be in pain, rather than not having fun and still having pain. (That's not to say, I never ask, 'Why am I doing this?' during a particularly painful warm-up stretch!) Circus involvement keeps low-grade depression, which is often lurking around my back door, at bay. People who haven't seen me for a while say I look good and I attribute that to a general sense of being more 'up' than feeling pulled down by life's problems. I have an outlet for gaining physical strength and flexibility, and for being creative at the same time. I have a place where I am affirmed and valued, not just for what I can do, but also for who I am. To have women whom I respect and admire believe in me makes even the tedious repeating of scenes in rehearsal worthwhile. A little praise from the director or trainer or someone who has seen the show doesn't go astray either!

Expanding horizons

Katrina Varian, Dunedin, New Zealand

Katrina Varian, MB ChB MGP, is a lecturer in the School of Occupational Therapy, Otago Polytechnic. She teaches in the area of health and disability, and has published research with women who have rheumatoid arthritis.

This article describes my experience of living with a stroke that significantly disabled me. I have chosen to focus on a tiny aspect of my life, that of how improving mobility has allowed me to venture out again, gradually re-engaging with the richness of life. I am a professional woman, aged 50, and in this account I look back over 20 years of disability, as well as alluding to current aspirations.

The perpetual change associated with living with a disability has a challenging and exciting quality. Growth springs from disability. I knew I might have a stroke in my late twenties, so when it happened I was able to have a positive view of reclaiming my abilities. At first it was hard work but progress was steady. From a wheelchair I began to walk again, first around the house and then the garden.

I live alone in a tiny house with a huge garden. It is the garden that has been the focus for my creativity since my stroke. I have always loved the outdoors. Just being outside with the sun on my face satisfied me at the beginning. My garden is really part of the Bush and the birds love it. My philosophy has been to garden in harmony with the Bush, cutting back or planting shrubs that contrast in colour, shape and texture. I see and interpret things differently now. I take in details, the colour of insects, small flowers, seed formations and other minutiae of nature that I've never noticed before. There is vitality all around me. It captures my attention. A new part of my brain has woken up!

Gradually I have become more adventurous, walking out into the world, first over the hill to the little port. I got to know the locals there much better and my circle of friends increased. After a few years, an adapted car meant I was able to take my dog, Basil, to the beach, and on other adventures. This really expanded our horizons. We loved to walk on the beach at low tide. I was able to rediscover the delight of lapping waves, cry of the seagulls and smell of the sea. I revelled in the wind on my face, burning sun and sand in my hair. Such sensations, after a period of loss, were a joy. I remember vividly a particular evening when we climbed a nearby headland. It is imprinted on my memory. I had climbed higher and higher, partly on my hands and knees. I knew I was pushing the boundaries. There were narrow ledges and steep drops, but the top flattened out to a small plateau. It was evening and the sky was changing hue. I knew that climbing down would be a challenge but also, deep within me, I knew that taking risks was the only way to grow. It is these experiences that have transformed me.

Again and again I have pushed out further from my comfort zone by taking risks. I now cox the local rowing four, an entirely new challenge: so close to the water I let it run through my fingers! I am dependent on people in some ways, but now there is more give and take. Although they lift me into the boat, they also trust my judgement, making me part of the team. Our journeys towing the boats have taken me further afield and on more co-operative endeavours. These undertakings have changed me: made me more daring. Starting with the garden, then to distant horizons, I have been through a transformation of recovery. Images in my mind from recent expeditions need to be expressed. I want to share the way I see things. It's my turn to create, to explore by photography. It is time I did the transforming.

Fun, challenges and endless surprises

Marley Critcher, Hunter Region, NSW, Australia

In the morning my two little dogs jump up on my bed and play until they wake me enough. They have an unquestioning trust that I will get up and feed them (one of them won't give up until I do). I love the simplicity of a dog's life: something to eat, someone to hug, a warm and safe place to live and something to run around and bark at with great passion. And this is how I see my life: each new day I see past the housework, the meals and any problems, and look forward with a passion to maybe fitting in some work with fibre.

I work full-time as a musician – and I love my work, but like all work it has responsibilities, deadlines and outcomes. The work I do with fibre has fun, challenges and endless surprises, especially when things turn out as I would have expected (this is the biggest surprise of all).

I have lived on my own since my husband died, and I am not plagued with loneliness like some because I am always eager to be getting on with what I am doing next. I am typically weaving or knitting project number 1, spinning wool for project number 2, dyeing the wool for project number 3 and preparing the wool to start project number 4. I consider that what I do is art. Amazingly, my house is not always in a mess! I do not want to be on my own for ever, but neither do I intend to compromise and settle for less than I deserve. I have a large group of friends with similar interests, and I am studying for a (two-year) certificate of spinning. This has led to me becoming involved in a group that takes part in an annual worldwide spinning and knitting competition, in which we shear a sheep, spin the wool and knit a jumper in eight hours or less, this is the best fun (last year we came fourth).

Over the last six years I have had about 20 dates; of those, only three of the guys had hobbies or interests besides their work. *All* the others had obvious drinking problems – the daughter of one man told me straight out that he was an alcoholic and to be careful; well, as we never got past the phone stage it was not a problem. I tell any prospective suitors that they have to phone me after 8.30 pm because of my work hours;

this is largely true, but makes it very easy to pick out who has the problems. I am not against alcohol. One time a guy asked me why I was seeking a partner when I already had a life!!! My answer to that is that you should be whole and fully functioning before inflicting yourself on someone else.

I recently got a reading from a clairvoyant who informed me that my life had taught me to be emotionally self-sufficient, and she is right. I have had a hard life, but I am happy in my own company, I love life, have never ever been bored, nor have I ever suffered depression.

I consider myself to be very life rich – I own my little house and car. I have two little dogs that trust me absolutely. I can play, listen to and write music, I have a great family and heaps of friends. I pass on my music knowledge to my students, and I have the passion of my hobby.

Thank goodness for my painting

Rita Wenberg, Albury, NSW, Australia

Also refer to the National Library of Australia (2001). Rita May Wenberg in 'Bringing Them Home' Oral history project, Canberra, Australia.

Before I took up painting – drawing,
                              I was going through same real bad
time, I just went on my own, to be on my own, I lost interest in everything, another word I lost interest in life.
            To me painting and drawing save my life, and mind,

When I am painting, you don't think of the bad time,
            to me I feel so peaceful looking at my work, I am in another world,
When I do landscape I feel as I am in the painting, it feel so nice

thank-goodness I love my painting, drawing.

While in Parramatta Girls Home,
I remember that I had a break-down, I was put into hospital part of the home, I suppose there was other things, but I can't remember.

Aboriginal!   I hate that name.
                         yes I still really haven't accepting, who I am realy,
            I am trying.

I lost interest in everything because of all the abuse I went through, cruely, you think things is going well, something alright come up.

I always think why did this happen me, I was just a child at the time, everything went wrong,
             of often think "why me"
only for my painting
                If I didn't have that, my mind start to think about what
happen to me, flash back.
             thank goodness for my Painting

A feeling of wholeness

Compiled by Eve Gray

Here are a few responses from women I asked to describe the effects a
creative activity had on them physically and/or mentally. The first two are
in a creative writing group and met once a week for five and eight years,
respectively. The group writes on the spot for about three hours, has published anthologies and other books, the members regularly win prizes (or
are commended) in competitions in poetry, short stories, etc. The degree
of commitment to writing varies, but commitment to the group, fellow
members, and the local community is fervent. They live within range of a
beautiful rural village and enjoy the camaraderie.

Ann

Not being a creative person, I found this difficult to answer.

Physically

Only thing I can think of is sewing – embroidery, tapestry, patchwork.
These all need a certain amount of concentration and force me to sit still.
Perhaps making a cake for family consumption at Christmas. Or creating
a new garden.

Mentally

Down by the creek there is the opportunity for contemplation and exploring the five senses through imagination.
I see the green willows on the opposite bank and flashes of flying colour
– in my mind this becomes shot silk,
sensuously wrapped around my body.
I hear the wind susurrating through the casuarinas, whispering to me
alone. I smell some light spindrift scent.
I taste the water which becomes wine.
I feel the fine sand through my fingers, warm as my lover's skin.

(I, Eve, then asked her to describe her feelings when engaged in a creative activity.)

> switched off mind . . . love it . . . contentment . . . satisfaction . . . achievement

Bette

Whether it comes from serving a well-cooked, well-presented meal for a special occasion, or a nourishing, filling meal to a hungry group, a sense of self-worth is achieved from doing or making something which is appreciated by others. It is the appreciation of others for your work that reinforces that sense of self-worth.

To make something – a quilt, a cushion or a poem to your own high standard gives a glow of well-being. Belonging to a group with similar interests stimulates the enthusiasm of each member of the group, and ideas can be shared and improved upon. Constructive criticism, friendship and laughter are shared, making each meeting a social time as well as a working time. Attending regular group sessions for any creative activity gives an escape when family and career are abandoned.

Jill

Eve introduces Jill: 'With the difficulty of suffering from attention deficit disorder, one participant, Jill, had to give up creative writing after chemotherapy; she believed her brain was affected. She also said as there was no feeling in her hands and feet, she took up spinning again as a type of therapy . . . at first just pulling wool apart into staples. Later, the hand, foot and eye co-ordination helped in rehabilitation. Also, she felt spinning had helped her recover more quickly following the second sessions of chemo.'

Jill commented, 'Spinning is like a type of meditation and it is very satisfying and calming.'

Julie

I weld, I write, therefore I am. Being born into a family that always 'did things', sitting around was a sin and there was no such thing as a couch potato in my childhood. I drew, painted, cut out and read endlessly, squirrelling away the gems of 'useless information', art appreciation and visual memories that I draw upon today.

Having left Sydney for the Hunter Valley, I joined the local TAFE's Rural Welding group in order to learn how to make farm implements. Originally, it was more of a cost-cutting exercise than a desire to 'create' things out of metal, but that soon changed. I found I loved steel in the way other friends loved wood. It's a bit of a fight, steel; so hard to cut, bend and shape without the right tools and techniques. This class offered space, a workshop full of big toys, and teachers willing to guide us through our projects. It was also full of fatherly blokes who offered assistance at every turn; initially, I arrived home with some terrific stuff but very little of it was my own work. The true joy of welding came when a teacher who was a 'closet sculptor' – a man who drew terrific twists, turns and swoops from ordinary strips of steel – inspired me to escape from the practicality of farm gates, hose reels and animal feeders in order to make the ornate gazebo I had dreamed about for years. Because of its size, my project was designed to be made in six separate panels in class, and then assembled at home with a portable welder.

I remember sitting in the sun on a patch of cleared ground, laying out dozens of scrolls made from cut-offs in class, wild tendrils of metal that were to become embellishments for the plain bandstand-style framework and, more exciting still, the tails of two peacocks displaying on each side of the 'doorway'. I also discovered the joy and frustration of using an oxytorch to cut out the eight metal sun faces and sculptured goats' heads that both decorated and hid the lumpy welds where the pitched roof met the walls of my hexagonal gazebo. I learnt heaps and had a lot of surprises before the decorative panels finally fell into place. Twisting and turning pieces of metal around in the dust made things 'happen'; the steel fell into shapes, designs and pictures I'd not previously thought of, and it was great to feel these structures changing and growing under my hands.

The curved steeple roof was a right bugger to control, and I needed the help of a strong neighbour to get the whole thing together at home. This project was definitely not a solo effort but it brought me a lot of satisfaction, friendship and trouble. Also, being totally unmathematical, it gave me a new sense of spacial recognition as the forms rose from the flat blueprint. It is the prettiest, most challenging (and certainly the largest) project I have ever undertaken; the truest translation and most concrete result of anything that had started in my head – and I often wonder now how I ever did it.

Writing gives me a much more fluctuating sense of satisfaction or wellbeing. It is far harder to measure if one has been 'successful' or not. It has a built-in stress factor and makes a most uneven graph. It's an itch to be scratched. A terrible need to escape into my own world. Amy Whiting wrote 'to find out what she thought' and I can really relate to that. It makes me rummage through my mind files, finds gaps only further research can fill, but it also leaves me feeling haggard, empty or totally blocked at times. When I have the odd success, publication or a competition win, I walk on air for 24 hours before the euphoria evaporates and then I feel strangely detached from it. It is not a monument to my imagination like the gazebo, even if it has been 'confirmed' by some outside 'judge'. It is a more fleeting satisfaction, like sex or cigarettes. The sort of 'hit' I imagine some people get from running or swimming. Writing is a dodgy way to find 'wellbeing' or 'satisfaction' but the desire to do it is certainly addictive.

Eve

When one is ill

- The rhythmic, lyrical nature of spinning allows the mind the freedom to ramble unfettered, and to switch off from any problems that beset it. The escape may be brief, but the respite gives one the strength to carry on and to cope.
- Writing, on the other hand, be it poetry or prose, tends to generate stress while one relives or recreates the emotions or tensions. Then comes the total obsessive absorption of trying to get it right and, finally, the absolute release and rush of pleasure when something is completed.

When one is not ill

- The craft of spinning is gratifying, satisfying and mesmeric. Like meditation, it takes us elsewhere and uses parts of the brain that are not used in everyday activities. It frees the brain for a different type of cerebral function. The finished product and its usefulness or beauty are a reward.
- Writing is a compulsion to create . . . perhaps like sculpting, painting, composing, etc. . . . there is a mass of impressions or beliefs inside needing to come out and be presented whole. I believe everyone is born creative, but that suppression (self or imposed) leads to aggression, discontent and 'unhealth'. Creativity gives the creator a feeling of wholeness – completing the cycle.

Creativity comes from love

Siobhan, Sound Minds, Battersea, London, UK

Often, when I lie awake, if the sun is shining and bright, it brings a positive feeling to me, which kind of inspires creative activity. But this isn't always the case. As a sufferer of bipolar disorder, I get really bad days of morose, dark deep depression – I get so low that nothing can help. Sometimes I may reach out for my art equipment as a means of therapy, to express just how bad, or depending on my mood, to express just how happy and glad I am to be alive in this wonderful world.

When I was a young girl, I must really have been very funny – a sort of harum scarum, almost a St Trinian's little convent schoolgirl, ordering around all my friends, to dance, sing and play act. And I was dead sure I was gonna be a choreographer or a Fantastic Actress. Dreaming my life away, perhaps often preventing my true creativity. But, creativity or the inspiration to be creative comes, for me, from the seasons, the natural world and natural wildlife, from my little daughter and all the fun stuff she says, and what children do, and, naturally, perhaps the most important thing that we all need in this life – well, love.

Falling in love, feeling love, in love with love, love of oneself, love for your friends and family. Love really inspires my creativity with no holds barred! I am inspired to paint or draw, write poetry or write songs. Some other days I just think, 'Oh, thank you God, my God, my Lord, this is the day that the Lord made so it is good,' and I'm glad to be living in it, no matter what I'm going through. Other days I might just think, 'Oh God, please help me, I can't cope, I can't go on, what will I do?' Somewhere, from someone, or something, eventually comes a glimmer of hope, which inspires my faith and my creativity too.

Sometimes after a hard day of drudgery and finding no enjoyment in my housework, or when nothing goes right, or I sense 'evil' at play, or I feel fear or that I am in real danger, I sometimes 'shout to the top' like Paul Weller sang about. I shout about the wrongness of things, the injustice of this hard life that we go through. I am subject to violence now and then in my marriage, and my partner drinks heavily and goes on and on, as well as having to put up with accusations of madness thrown at me. Mad – why shouldn't I be mad, or get mad? Get mad, get even, yeah. Anyway, all sorts of personal dramas that I go through often help me to write or paint, or draw or play-act or dance. My writing sways from hopeful sweetness to dreadful, doom-laden trouble. The depths of London meanness, and the sudden charm of a kind smile, or a plea for help that is responded to – just once in a while. Hope, love. These would be better inspirations for all, not just for me.

Conclusion

While I am not attempting to draw conclusions from the above contributions about the success or value of creative activities, what is obvious is that all of the accounts do, in one way or another, express a highly valued involvement, and all demonstrate a belief that there are benefits to be obtained from that involvement.

CHAPTER 8

'Integrating the firelight of creativity': an evolving practice of creativity-based groupwork for health and well-being

SALLY DENSHIRE

Introduction

> [When I returned from overseas] I did some corporeal mime and a lot of dance and things – for expressive not performative reasons. Then I saw the Children's Hospital job and applied for that. My practice there was with young people – teenagers who came to hospital repeatedly and I seemed to have this strong drive to make this hospital as a territory – better for them. So I did a lot of groupwork with young people – got to know them really well – my practice was very relational . . . I was very much WITH them as a youth worker would be – I worked very informally, was very anti the clinical view and did a lot of creative work with them about finding their own voices and in parallel I was finding mine. (Denshire and Ryan, 2001, p. 155)

The 'Youth Arts Program' at the Children's Hospital involved both young people and arts workers in processes of 'creative exchange' (Denshire, 1993, p. 23). Generating creative possibilities together like this fostered a sense of shared humanity between us, rather than relating to one another based on professional distance. The process of reciprocal creation and participation was as important as the finished product. Indeed, if practitioners are to facilitate creative potential in others, then they most likely need to participate actively in the creative world themselves, as I describe above, in reflections from my life-writing.

Opportunities for creative expression that utilize craft, art and everyday creativity enable humans to communicate their individuality and to learn about the world by experimentation and the production of occupational artefacts (Cynkin and Robinson, 1990). Engaging in creative occupations, using a range of media to portray lived experiences, alone and with others, may be particularly necessary for humans to survive and flourish in potentially alienating environments.

148

The creativity-based groupwork approaches described here have come from my experiences with young people in hospital and, more recently, with occupational therapy students. Also, when my children were small, I facilitated childbirth education groups with parents-to-be, and, as a new graduate, in collaboration with psychiatric nurses and social workers, I co-led a programme of groups on the admission ward of a large psychiatric hospital, in the days when such institutions were more commonplace. I have been part of ongoing psychodrama groups and community arts projects such as 'Theatre Reaching Environments Everywhere' (TREE).

In this way, my collaborative experiences of groupwork have spanned more than 25 years, from the delivery of creative activities programmes with teenagers in hospital to starting up and co-ordinating a cross-disciplinary groupwork service, and establishing and researching a children's hospital youth arts programme. Now, I continue to use creativity-based groupwork in the education of student occupational therapists. They exhibit their everyday creative artefacts and photographs in collaborations with photography students from the School of Visual and Performing Arts.

This chapter begins with an overview of literature on contemporary contexts for creativity-based groupwork, successful art and health projects, groupwork and creativity-based approaches, the facilitator's 'imaginative self', youth creativity and a sense of positive health, and creative arts projects as rites of passage. An account of the exhibition of everyday creative artifacts by student occupational therapists follows. The values that figure in this narrative have emerged from deep reflection on my professional and personal group experiences, and they support my approach to creativity-based groupwork. Finally, suggestions are made for incorporating these health-promoting approaches in the planning of our future health services.

Creativity-based groupwork approaches

Contemporary contexts for creativity-based groupwork

At the beginning of the twenty-first century, contradictions posed and imposed by forces of globalization confront us. On one hand, we encounter the dissolution of economic boundaries and the erosion of cultural differences through the impact of mass communication and information networks. On the other, we see an increasing emergence of groups and communities asserting their differences and separateness in a bid to maintain a sense of identity and establish themselves as sites of resistance (McDermott, 2002).

The sense of emotional, physical and social well-being that group participation brings is reported anecdotally and in the literature (Tindale et al., 1998; Corey, 2000). Our experiences of working with groups occur within a globalized world. In this way contemporary groupwork impacts upon, and is shaped by, this broader context.

Successful art and health projects

The relationship between creativity and healing is well established (Adamson, 1984; Yeats, 1993; Allen, 1996). In this chapter, I use the term 'healing' in the broad sense to mean the recovery of wholeness and healthful restoration. People who are involved in art-making through creativity-based groups may be essentially healthy, chronically ill or simply facing turning points in their lives. Engagement in art-making during groups and festivals can promote a sense of spiritual wholeness, identity and fulfilment that can be health-enhancing for the participants (VicHealth, 2003).

Documentation of the effectiveness of arts programmes based in healthcare settings in Australia and overseas is becoming more common (*see* Confetti, 1986; MacDonald, 1990; Gilman, 1992; Marsden, 1993; Buckland, 1994; Marsden and Thiele, 2000). For example, Opperman and Dreyfus (1996) discussed the empowering effect for service users in the maternity and aged care sections of an urban hospital where they had transformed age-specific spaces by using photography and ceramics. Fowler Smith (1996) outlined the positive impact on the health of disturbed adolescents from collaboratively designing an outdoor courtyard in a psychiatric ward. There are further examples in Chapter 9.

Groupwork and creativity-based approaches

The interdisciplinary, groupwork literature has focused on issues of leadership and co-leadership, group processes, group dynamics and on planning, evaluating and intervening in groups (Bundey et al., undated). Bion (1961) and Yalom (1975) have discussed practices of group psychotherapy, and writers such as Douglas (1976, 1978) and Konopka (1963) have established a foundation for groupwork practice in social work. In occupational therapy, Finlay (1993) and Howe and Schwartzberg (1986) have discussed general principles for groupwork.

When we turn to creativity-based approaches in contemporary society, 'play' appears to have been undervalued (Vandenberg and Kielhofner, 1982). Miller and Fox (1988, p. 3) defined creativity as the 'forgotten link in occupational therapy'. However, more recently, Cynkin and Robinson (1990) and Breines (1995) highlighted the use of creative arts in occupational therapy to promote health and well-being. Creativity

psychotherapy (Hurst, 1988) can offer relevant approaches to both practitioners and participants involved in processes of creativity and
transpersonal healing.

Sue Jennings (1986) is an experienced drama therapist who has written
extensively on creative drama in groupwork. Liebmann (1986) has written
about art therapy for groups. The inspirational Chilean drama-therapist,
Aldo Gennaro, with whom I have had the pleasure of working, used theatre training and improvisation to empower young adults living with
intellectual handicaps to take their place in the world. His work culmin-
ated in a public performance at the Sydney Opera House (Noonan, 1980).

A facilitator's 'imaginative self'

Fiona McDermott (2002) theorized groupwork practice by interrogating
group facilitators about their ways of thinking and feeling. Her focus on
using metaphor as a conceptual tool acknowledges the imaginative self
that groupworkers access in practice and the metaphors we rely on to
conceptualize practice. The imaginative self sparks our symbolic thinking
as part of everyday problem-solving. An emphasis on imagination and
metaphor is particularly relevant to groupwork approaches that are
grounded in the creativity of those involved.

We can understand metaphor as thinking of one thing in terms of
another. For example, when art student Michaelie Crawford christened a
project 'Art Injection' in 1991, she was using a metaphor that compared
art-making with an instrument that introduces something into the body:
an injection. My interpretation of this metaphor is that it communicates
the healing power of art-making in a surprising way, by making an unlike-
ly comparison between expression and medical intervention. I recall the
cake at the launch being in the shape of an artist's palette pierced with
syringes.

In the project, young people in hospital and art students collaborated
on sculptures such as 'Nil by mouth' and 'Giant doctor', made from
crutches and drip trays, and other recycled hospital equipment that had
previously been used during a young person's medical treatment.
Displaying these sculptures throughout the hospital during postgraduate
week provided a tangible starting point for developing more meaningful
communication around sensitive issues of compliance and power
between young people and their healthcare providers.

Our values and beliefs are carried in the metaphors we use (Denshire,
2002a). For example, another metaphor, 'integrating the firelight of creativity', which psychodramatist Stephanie Hurst suggested was one of the
tasks of an occupational therapist, appeals to my imagination because of

its alchemical symbolism and because of its ambiguity, which leaves the meanings of 'integrating' and 'firelight of creativity' open to the interpretation of the reader.

This metaphor implies that energy or a spark transmitted in the creative act keeps fires burning. Fire was an ancient symbol in alchemy, the mediaeval form of chemistry that tried to find ways of changing all metals into gold. This firelight does not appear to be owned; rather, my understanding is that it fuels a common energy that can be drawn on.

McDermott (2002) explained that metaphor is central to our capacity to construct meaning. As groupworkers, we engage with the lived experiences of leader and participants, with the poetic and the felt. We express our thoughts, ideas and values by using metaphors. These poetic and imaginative responses are our attempts, as groupworkers, to make sense of practice. In this way, when we think 'group', we are simultaneously thinking 'metaphor'. We engage our imaginative selves in groups, particularly in facilitating creative arts projects such as creating storyboards for cartoons, or when we brainstorm project ideas with a group, or map concepts for play-building.

Viewing groups as sites for construction and reconstruction of meaning brings together theory and practice, and points towards post-modern understandings of the world. Post-modern groupwork practice deals with uncertainty in interactions, deconstructs language and symbols, explores the possibilities of change and re-definition, and offers us opportunities to experience and explore our subjectivities with others (Parton and Marshall, 1998; as cited in McDermott, 2002). In this way, post-modern groupwork proceeds from recognition that the intersubjective context of the group can be a site for the construction and reconstruction of meaning. In other words, people may come to understand, control, reframe and develop their experiences by expressing themselves in groups (McDermott, 2002).

Youth creativity and a sense of positive health

Adolescence is a period of complex changes in physical growth and maturation, and of transition from childhood dependency to adult autonomy. During this phase, young people are struggling to establish their personal and sexual identity, and a sense of self-esteem and competence. It is also a time to develop satisfactory interpersonal relationships, increasing independence and an ability to cope with both needs and potentials (Dr. L. Henricks, personal communication, May, 1983).

Youth creativity emerges as a philosophy of approach when developing holistic health services with young people. It is derived from values found in youth-specific occupational therapy (Denshire, 1985), community arts (Kelly, 1984), youth health initiatives (Bennett, 1985; Peppard et al., 1988) and feminism (Hamlin et al., 1992) and seems to be related to feelings of positive health. These values are expanded upon under the heading, 'Values underlying creativity-based approaches' later in this chapter.

Franzkowiak (1984) outlined a model of positive health that can be regarded as a goal for the young person on reaching adulthood. Positive health involves the capacity to communicate and express oneself, and to create or change oneself and one's environment in a positive way. It also includes the ability to accommodate to the pain and problems of life in a peaceful way, instead of projecting oneself aggressively. The healthy person is able to realize potential for growth and fulfilment, for personal development and freedom. The opportunity and ability to join in and contribute to the local environment and community may be distinguished as basic characteristics of positive health.

Creative arts projects as rites of passage

The increasing orientation of adolescents towards social contacts outside their families makes them organize in peer groups and subcultures. These subcultures, as a whole, constitute the youth cultures of a modern society. Their function is to give young people the space to act out their generational concerns collectively and to work out successful ways to finish their 'passage of status' into the dominant adult culture (Brake, 1980).

In most primitive and some advanced societies, groups are formed for warriors, or young people at puberty, or adults who are at the same stage of life, who face the same problems and have similar tasks ahead. Group participation provides peers and mutual support. These groups are settings in which to master the activities, tools and rituals that are needed to cross from one developmental phase to the next in a given society (van Gennep, 1960; Kitzinger, 1977; Mahdi et al., 1987). The current lack of rituals in society may leave people with a hunger that may be satisfied through meaningful group participation.

A young person's creative development may be affected, depending on gender, by societal messages about the desirability, or otherwise, of self-expression and creativity. In the hospital environment, however, this was rarely an issue. The pressures at school to conform to gendered behaviours did not seem to apply to young people in hospital (L. Croft-Piggin, personal communication, September, 2003). The imagination necessary for art-making usually remains unaffected during experiences of illness.

A focus is emerging on public and community health approaches that are intended to enhance well-being. As part of this shift, dedicated creative arts projects can augment the natural groupings that form spontaneously to accomplish rites of passage within our post-industrial society. The following account of an exhibition of everyday creative artifacts by students who are in the process of becoming occupational therapists illustrates this point well.

'From me and my piece to us and our exhibition'

Rituals of professional socialization

In the third-year experiential subject 'Occupation: Experiences and Opportunities' (in Occupational Therapy at Charles Sturt University, Albury, NSW, Australia), humans are understood as 'occupational beings' (Clark et al., 1996, p. 374). Humans have occupational needs to be productive, to create artefacts and to experience leisure in conducive environments such as domestic spaces or workshops, and in alienating environments such as hospitals or prisons. The subject helps students to gain practice insights as part of their professional socialization, by doing projects they have selected themselves to enhance a sense of well-being through occupations such as making furniture, photography and toy-making.

Making a constructive, expressive piece

Working in wood, metal, textiles, film and mixed media, students spent 12 hours or more making a constructive, expressive piece of their own choosing, based on a similar assignment designed by occupational therapy academics, Cynkin and Robinson (1990). Reflecting on their personal experiences of the creative process enriches the experiential repertoire used in occupational therapy practice, adding to their store of experiential knowledge.

Getting ready for the exhibition

Students are able to make the link between personal creativity and the practice of occupational therapy in health settings through participation in this exhibition. They certainly identified working in groups to prepare for the exhibition as an important learning experience. Groups worked on curation and hanging, cataloguing, publicity, signage, catering, hosting, documentation and an opening ceremony. The students regarded their exhibition as the culmination of three years of study.

Opening night

As Belinda Henning, our Master of Ceremonies, said on opening night: 'Working in groups to put all this together taught us all about planning, problem-solving, co-operation and diplomacy! It moved the project from me and my piece, to us and our exhibition.'

Members of the audience commented that seeing this range of constructive, expressive pieces increased their understanding of occupational therapists as people and as practitioners. Further reflection on the descriptions of each piece extended an understanding of the connections between practitioners' personal and professional life spaces as necessary for congruent practice in the twenty-first century (Denshire, 2002b).

From public space to cyberspace

Thanks to the sustained collaboration of students, subject co-ordinator and educational designers, the exhibition is now on the internet. You can judge for yourself! Visit our online exhibition (Charles Sturt University, 1998) at: www.csu.edu.au/faculty/health/cmhealth/OT/OT.html

There has been an evolution from a literal to a virtual environment, from public space to cyberspace. With the existence of the website, our public exhibition is now international, rather than local.

The group as a site for meaning construction

The educational rationale underlying the original exhibition was that students would create works that linked their personal creativity with their professional practice, and that staging an exhibition would facilitate teamwork and encourage reflection. The move to cyberspace has taken this one step forward; the 'staging' of the exhibition on the internet moves it from an ephemeral space to relative permanency, from a local event to an international stage, and the web medium provides an opportunity for further reflection, not just by the current group of students, but by future students, as shown in the following comments by students' reviews of the site:

> In showcasing the creative skills of future occupational therapists it demonstrates that creativity is not a unique gift, rather, the potential for creativity exists within us all. (Glenn Becher, unpublished website review)

> . . . a clear example of the importance of creativity, not only within the profession but to the individual. The site shows how creativity is applied or expressed differently according to the individual interpretation of the concept. The Creative Links site also demonstrated the inherent place of creativity in society today. (Billie-Jo Smythe, unpublished website review)

A few students felt uncomfortable with the way self-expression was emphasized in the subject. They felt safer with techno-rational approaches to practice, and described the site content as 'primitive' or 'backward-looking'.

By bringing theory and practice together, the exhibition draws on constructivist theory, which emphasizes active learning using groupwork, sharing ideas, knowledge and reflection, and learning through experience. This collaboration promotes the idea of a partnership between client and practitioner, which is so essential to problem-solving as we enter the twenty-first century.

More recently, as part of their professional socialization, third-year students curated two photographic exhibitions with the accompanying catalogues *Life Reflected in Art: Occupation Reflected in Photography* (Harrower et al., 2000) and *Beneath: Reflections on Occupation* (McGregor et al., 2001), in collaboration with photography students from the School of Visual and Performing Arts.

Values underlying creativity-based approaches

The underlying values that support my approach to creativity-based groupwork are creative expression, peer-group participation, experiential learning, well-being through doing, place-making and cross-disciplinary collaboration. I discuss the significance of each one in turn in this part of the chapter, drawing on my writings about the 'Youth Arts Program'.

Making opportunities for creative expression: 'the need for expression that comes from being trapped'

The 'Youth Arts Program' was developed in 1984 to meet the health and maturational needs of young people in an Australian hospital. The participants in the programme were young people, aged between 12 and 20, who experienced repeated and prolonged hospitalization at a time of life when their struggle for autonomy was at its peak. Their need for developmental space was very real, and it was necessary for their service providers and researchers to comprehend that.

The establishment of the programme acknowledged the participants as 'occupational beings'. These young people were active, speaking subjects who were able to do some things they found personally meaningful, rather than always having to be passive patients lying in bed. The programme provided opportunities for enjoyment through creativity, and a collective voice within the hospital environment. These young people created masks, video art and computer-generated images, giant board games, radio documentaries, stories, poetry, sculpture and cultural events. The arts projects took place around the wards, corridors and grounds in a paediatric teaching hospital, occurring at the symbolic intersection of youth culture and hospital culture.

Comments by young people on paediatric wards, prior to the opening of the adolescent ward, indicate the perceived value of earlier projects:

'We got a chance to do something that teenagers would like to do instead of doing things that children do.'

Since opening in 1987, the adolescent ward has been the main site of creative occupation, and here, positive changes to both the built environment and the social environment have been evident. When asked to comment on the personal relevance of the 'Youth Arts Program', one of the main participants, who was living with cystic fibrosis, put it this way: 'There is a need for expression that comes from being trapped inside a world of unescapable sickness and continuous hospitalization.'

With relocation of the hospital imminent, it became urgent to capture the essence of the 'Youth Arts Program', which is unique in an Australian hospital setting, by creating a permanent, accessible record of finished works. The programme inspires many chronically ill young people, has produced a variety of challenging works, generated media attention, and continues to achieve local and international recognition for youth arts practice in a healthcare setting. These young people have created a range of pieces in collaboration with successive youth arts teams of health workers, arts workers and students from different disciplines. The archival materials comprise original two- and three-dimensional works, audio-visual and print media, and records of creativity-based group sessions. Most of these works were, by their very nature, ephemeral, so photographic documentation on slides was necessary. The archive was completed in July 1994, and is housed in a cabinet, painted with aerosol art specially commissioned from a young artist living with a chronic illness. Storage on CD-ROM of entire archives such as this is recommended.

Participating with peers: 'the participation was the best'

Young people in hospital who were involved in 'Telling Tales', a three-day storytelling workshop where participants made their own slide–tape sequence before the opening of the adolescent ward, have commented favourably on the value of participation with other young people:

> The participation was the best. I found it very interesting meeting other people my age, as it was extremely dull on the ward with children half my age, with only schoolwork and TV to keep me company. 'Telling Tales' was great fun and I got a lot out of it.

Participants in the film-making project over the school holidays made reference to what they perceived as the value of 'doing':

> We made a film at the Adolescent Medical Unit, and that was something like adults do, and we got a chance to do something that teenagers would like to do instead of doing things that children do.

For a practitioner working with young people, much of the work simply involved 'being there'. As Hirsch (as cited in Silverstein, 1973, p. 107) described, 'we need to reach out to [young people] in their natural groupings and by joining them we can intervene constructively'.

Young people could do a range of activities at the bedside or in the youth centre. Rather than replicate the cultureless features of hospital life, the youth centre at the Adolescent Medical Unit communicates a 'press' (Barris, 1982) for participation, informality and choice, by the presence of artefacts such as a comfortable, second-hand lounge-suite, floor cushions, rock-music posters, a radio tuned to a popular station, partly finished wall-paintings, personal possessions, space-invaders and a pool-table. Here, young people congregate, and can get involved in low-key recreation or arts projects such as 'Your First Flat', a series of group meetings for young people setting up house.

The extent to which a teenager can participate in a healthcare setting needs some consideration. At 'The Door', a multi-service youth centre in New York, which I visited in 1983, roles for young people included reception, accompanying others, acting as a host or guide, advocacy, devising resources and teaching creative skills, health education, advising, planning and evaluation. Youth in these roles provided a 'barometer' for a service. Young people, as members of a youth advisory board, were able to contribute to policy formulation. Resource staff are needed to co-ordinate training experiences, develop roles and job descriptions for youth, and facilitate groups to reflect on experiences. Young people in these roles also need space of their own within the centre.

Principles of experiential learning: 'create a place where the learning rises up'

In order to facilitate experiential learning about creative occupation, the exhibition process was handed over to the students to interpret according to their own interests and desires. As the educator, I remained responsible for the final outcome of the project. This emphasis on individual and collective, creative expression by student occupational therapists paralleled the other youth arts projects I have facilitated. Participants experienced a stronger sense of identity, self-esteem and belonging through creative expression in these projects. Some chose to have education and professional socialization as their goal rather than healing and recovery.

Now, as an educator, I can reflect on the application of experiential learning to creativity-based groupwork:

> Creativity and healing is really the heart of my practice. I founded the Youth Arts Program and now, in my present role as an academic, that transfers to creativity and learning and that's what I recognise and bring out in my

students. I find peer learning and working with groups in a relational way is a very satisfying means to create a learning environment. Where students continue their learning in a number of modes not only using text. Where the students' voices are very much uppermost and I just create a place where the learning rises up. (Denshire and Ryan, 2001, p. 156)

Given that creativity-based group sessions with young people in hospital often took place in the youth centre across the road from the hospital, perhaps the youth-specific occupational therapist was regarded as someone who took young people to an unseen place, hidden from the gaze of ward staff. (Another staff member has referred to me as a 'Pied Piper'.) The emphasis on peer groupwork and creative occupation was not well understood by some medical and nursing staff in the early years of the programme, but gradually this changed as the 'underground practice' became more public.

Feel a sense of well-being through doing: 'we used to do lots of stuff with clay'

My own sense of well-being seems to come, in part, from childhood experiences while on holiday with a naturally occurring peer group, as described in my life-writing:

> We used to do lots of stuff with clay. There was a rock called Doctor's Rock that had these sandstone benches on it. It was an enormous rock as big as this room and we would climb on top of it and spend all day doing this stuff using clay from the bush. So where we went on holidays was very much a very free sort of space. Being there was about running around with this big throng of other kids and having all these adventures, playing all these imaginary games, and then collecting the shells as sort of memories of our holiday place that I would bring back home in a cardboard box. (Denshire and Ryan, 2001, p. 154)

Earlier I have argued, 'participation is health-enhancing in and of itself, a way of empowering young people, recognizing their capabilities and a means of changing the health system to make it more responsive to young people' (Denshire, 1984). Youth participation establishes adolescents and adults as partners and provides a foundation based on strengths and competence for working together. Further, this action acknowledges what Eisenstein and others refer to as the 'authority of experience' of the teenager and the validity of experiential learning as part of a positive concept of health (Denshire, 1984, p. 6).

Programme participants were often asked to evaluate each project at the time it was happening. The following comment is typical of the way young people value doing personally meaningful things:

The best thing about 'Telling Tales' was that we did positive things in our spare time like getting organized, making up slides of story pictures (similar to a movie), making friends and just having a good time.'

Space and place matter: 'painting all the walls and painting all the things'

Territory being vital to teenagers, the opening of a 10-bed adolescent ward was a major breakthrough for young people and their families who were 'regular customers' at hospital. Now that the hospital has relocated to Westmead, the expanded ward continues to serve the medical and surgical needs of hospitalized teenagers in an atmosphere compatible with their growth and psychosocial development. Having their own ward ensures adolescents a real place in the scheme of things. The establishment of such a ward is tangible acknowledgement that teenage patients support each other, and receive better and more comprehensive care when they are grouped together.

The archival data revealed the space and place dimensions of creative occupation as recurring themes that had significance for young people in hospital. With the opening of the adolescent ward in 1987, young people finally had a dedicated space within the hospital. Earlier arts projects, such as 'The Ward Game' and the 'Great Escape 2' film project, had conveyed the pressing need for such youth-specific space. In the following speech, given at the film première, one participant spoke on behalf of other teenagers about the importance of 'place':

> Our film is based on teenagers having a ward of their own, no matter what sort of sickness they've got. The film is based on teenagers organizing their own ward. This is how we made our movie. We started off last week by watching other movies to collect ideas for our movie. We were taught how to operate cameras, lighting, directing and how to do make up, while we were working out how to co-operate with each other. Our story was drawn on paper first. This is called a storyboard.

Hospitalization represents a major crisis for adolescents. It heightens body-image concerns, causes separation from family and friends, places restriction on mobility, invades privacy and enforces dependency at a time when the struggle for autonomy is at its peak. In a hospital geared, primarily, to the medical needs of sick babies and young children, ill and injured adolescents face special difficulties, especially when they are scattered throughout the wards solely on the basis of diagnosis.

The hospital setting demands of adolescents a passive and vulnerable role, in which feelings of helplessness are exacerbated. Entering a hospital means entering a different culture. The idea of youth participation can be politically sensitive in medical settings because it flies in the face of the dominant organizational culture. In some sense, involvement in creative occupation offered these young people a place within the culture of the hospital as well as in the world outside. Acting on the environment like this seems to develop a sense of identity and a shared awareness of youth culture to counteract what Clarke (1976) refers to as 'hospital shock'. Hospital shock can be understood as a kind of culture shock, where the sense of personal space and the presence of familiar ritual and everyday objects are disrupted by the unfamiliar culture of hospital life. By engaging in creative occupation, young people stake their own place in the social space within the hospital. One participant living with a chronic illness vividly described how the space was transformed:

> Boring old black wall, looking at that all the time sends your mind go crazy. Just a white ward and curtains, brown curtains. I think that made you sick just waking up and looking at that all the time. As soon as *Art Injection* came around, that all changed, like they were painting all the walls and painting all the things.

In this way, creative occupation in arts projects converted the space on an adolescent ward into a place of young people. The distinction between space and place, in this context, is a subtle one. An adolescent space has the potential to become a youth-specific place of territory and ownership. This is a place where the occupants have moved in and 'put their stamp'.

Cross-disciplinary collaboration: 'working together on projects in a multimodal way'

Arts workers from a range of disciplines were more often generalists working together on projects in a multimodal way. We used networking to collaborate with different parts of the hospital community to devise and exhibit creative work, such as video projects, radio documentaries or magazines. The 'Youth Arts Program' had a community-arts, collective-voice perspective, rather than a focus on psychodynamic art therapy or on professional art practice.

However, debates about whether arts workers needed to be specialists or generalists have been ongoing. Although the occupational therapists involved in the programme were generalists, some of the artists had in-depth skills in particular media. Film-maker, Laura Hastings-Smith, took the view that 'through an exchange of those skills, which as a professional artist are linked to the art community and the wider society, young people have access to quality instruction' (Hastings-Smith, 1988, p. 95). Certainly, a thorough understanding by the artist-in-residence of the medium in which the young artist has chosen to work may facilitate the completion and exhibition of projects.

Creativity theory that distinguishes between 'special talent' creativity and 'self-actualized' creativity (Miller, 1992) is useful in understanding the devaluation of community arts initiatives, by certain sectors of the art world, due to the tendency to work in generalist, ordinary ways, rather than striving to attain fine-arts expertise (Connell, 1983; Heks, 1991). Such generalist ways of working characterized the intended role of a designated creative-resources co-ordinator.

Ways to integrate creativity-based groupwork

The following priorities for creativity-based groupwork are suggested for a contemporary approach to designing and delivering a truly integrated health service.

Creative expression

Build in permanent opportunities for all sorts of creative expression by people using the health service. Ensure the availability of skilled, talented staff, attractive facilities and materials, and, most important, engender an organizational culture that promotes the value of creativity-based approaches that, often, can be unconventional (and therein lies their richness).

Peer-group participation

Promote peer-group participation, not only among young people but also across the lifespan, by offering ongoing group and community experiences to the people who use the service, rather than having an exclusive focus on the individual.

Experiential learning

Use the principles of experiential learning in the delivery of creativity-based groups by encouraging people to participate actively with a range of media, followed by reflection on the experience.

Well-being through doing

Foster a sense of well-being in the people involved in programmes by ensuring that the available creativity-based, group projects are of high calibre and ongoing, rather than short-lived, pilot projects 'lurching' from short-term grant to short-term grant.

Space and place matter

Acknowledge the importance of space and place in site-specific projects by giving participants the option to personalize and 'put their stamp on' the particular spaces in which they are working. It means sharing power. It means allowing this to happen, and welcoming the cultural changes in the organization!

Working together

Encourage cross-disciplinary collaboration by providing sufficient funding for a fully resourced team of workers, from a range of different backgrounds, to work together in complementary ways, to plan, lead and evaluate creativity-based group programmes.

Conclusion

This chapter makes explicit some of the values and beliefs that have shaped my professional approaches to creativity-based groupwork over the last 25 years. Whenever we uncover the assumptions, beliefs and values that underpin how a particular group programme operates, then the theory that underlies the practice can emerge (McDermott, 2002). I have used processes of writing and reflection to articulate the value of creative expression, peer-group participation, experiential learning, well-being through doing, place-making and cross-disciplinary collaboration, in my work with young people.

As creativity-based workers, we need to 'integrate the firelight of creativity' to fuel our personal and professional lives in, what is often, the cold, hard light of economic rationalism. Then we can develop congruent ways to support and evaluate creativity-based projects. We need to cite congruent evidence from health-enhancing programmes, such as artistic product, creators' feedback and practitioners' reflections, to ensure that creativity-based groups survive, and indeed flourish, as integral parts of truly responsive health services. I trust my reflections will serve as useful maps to refer back to, as you explore the rich and fertile terrain of creativity-based groupwork.

Acknowledgements

I would like to pay tribute to the inspiring participants, co-leaders, colleagues and mentors I have had the pleasure of working with over the years. Thank you all!

References

Adamson ELC. Art as Healing. London: Coventure, 1984.

Allen P. Art is a Way of Knowing. London: Shambala, 1996.

Barris R. Environmental interactions: an extension of the model of occupation. American Journal of Occupational Therapy 1982; 36: 637–44.

Bennett DL. Adolescent Health in Australia. Sydney: Australian Medical Association, 1985.

Bion WR. Experiences in Groups. London: Tavistock Publications, 1961.

Brake M. The Sociology of Youth Culture and Youth Subcultures. London: Routledge & Kegan Paul, 1980.

Breines EB. Occupational Therapy Activities from Clay to Computers. Philadelphia, PA: FA Davis, 1995.

Buckland A. Art Injection: Youth Arts in Hospital. Camperdown, NSW, Australia: Royal Alexandra Hospital for Children, 1994.

Bundey C, Cullen J, Denshire L, Grant J, Norfor J, Nove T. Group Leadership. Sydney, Australia: NSW Department of Health, undated.

Charles Sturt University. Creative Links 1998. (Accessed 8 May 2004: www.csu.edu.au/faculty/health/cmhealth/OT/OT.html)

Clarke A. Hospital Shock. Dunedin, NZ: Mediaprint Services, 1976.

Clark F, Ennevor BL, Richardson PL. A grounded theory of techniques for occupational story telling and occupational story making. In: Zemke R, Clark F (eds), Occupational Science: The Evolving Discipline. Philadelphia, PA: FA Davis, 1996; 373–92.

Confetti D. The Side Effects Manual of Theatre Games and Role Plays for Youth. Sydney, Australia: Commonwealth National Health Promotion Program, 1986.

Connell B. Democratising culture. Meanjin 1983; 3: 295–307.

Corey G. Theory and Practise of Group Counseling (fifth edition). Pacific Grove, CA: Brookes/Cole, 2000.

Cynkin S, Robinson AM. Occupational Therapy and Activities Health: Toward Health Through Activities. Boston, MA: Little, Brown, 1990.

Denshire S. The Shape and Impact of Youth Participation in Health. Working paper prepared for Study Group on Young People and Health for All by the Year 2000. Geneva, Switzerland: World Health Organization, 1984.

Denshire S. Normal spaces in abnormal places: the significance of environment in occupational therapy with hospitalised teenagers. Australian Occupational Therapy Journal 1985; 32: 142–9.

Denshire S. Work of art: occupational analysis of a children's hospital youth arts programme. Youth Studies Australia 1993; 12: 18–24.

Denshire S. Metaphors we live by: ways of imagining practice. Qualitative Research Journal 2002a; 2: 28–46.

Denshire S. Reflections on the confluence of personal and professional. Australian Occupational Therapy Journal 2002b; 49: 212–16.

Denshire S, Ryan S. Using autobiographical narrative and reflection to link personal and professional domains. In: Higgs J, Titchen A (eds), Professional Practice in Health, Education and the Creative Arts. Oxford: Blackwell, 2001; 149–60.

Douglas T. Groupwork Practice. London: Tavistock, 1976.

Douglas T. Basic Groupwork. London: Tavistock, 1978.

Finlay L. Groupwork in Occupational Therapy. London: Chapman & Hall, 1993.

Fowler Smith J. Place, Space and Object Relations: The Making of an Outdoor Hospital Space for Psychotic and/or Suicidal Adolescents. Paper presented at the Intersections Conference, University of NSW, Australia, 1996.

Franzkowiak P. Health Promotion for Youth in the European Region: Basic Philosophy and Innovative Strategies. Working paper prepared for Study Group on Young People and Health for All by the Year 2000. Geneva, Switzerland: World Health Organization, 1984.

van Gennep A. The Rites of Passage (trans. MB Vizedom and GL Caffee). Chicago, IL: University of Chicago, 1960.

Gilman R. Community animation. In Context 1992; 4: 16–21.

Hamlin RB, Loukas KM, Froelich J, Macrae N. Feminism: an inclusive perspective. American Journal of Occupational Therapy 1992; 46: 967–70.

Harrower K, Ryan H, Steinberg A. Life Reflected in Art: Occupation Reflected in Photography. Exhibition catalogue. Albury, NSW, Australia: Occupational Therapy Programme, Charles Sturt University, 2000.

Hastings-Smith L. The Role of the Artist in Health Care Settings. Paper presented at the New Universals: Adolescent Health and A Time of Change, Sydney, NSW, Australia, 1988.

Heks R. Interview with Deborah Mills, Director of the Community Cultural Development Unit. Artlink 1991; 10: 49–52.

Howe M, Schwartzberg SL. A Functional Approach to Group Work in Occupational Therapy. Baltimore, MA: Lippincott, Williams & Wilkins, 1986.

Hurst S. The Occupational Therapist Integrates the Firelight of Creativity. Paper presented at the Australian Association of Occupational Therapists, 15th Federal Conference, National Perspective, Sydney, NSW, Australia, 1988.

Jennings S. Creative Drama in Group-work. Oxford: Winslow Press, 1986.

Kelly O. Storming the Citadels, Community Arts and the State. London: Comedia, 1984.

Kitzinger S. Education and Counselling for Childbirth. London: Cassell & Collier McMillan, 1977.

Konopka G. Social Group Work: A Helping Process. Englewood Cliffs, NJ: Prentice-Hall, 1963.

Liebmann M. Art Therapy for Groups: A Handbook of Themes, Games and Exercises. London: Croom Helm, 1986.

McDermott F. Inside Group-work: A Guide to Reflective Practice. Sydney, Australia: Allen & Unwin, 2002.

MacDonald D. The hospice world view: healing versus recovery. American Journal of Hospice and Palliative Care 1990; September/October: 39–45.

McGregor K, Nixon H, Harding M, Manton A, Pidgeon F, Grakini N. Beneath: Reflections on Occupation. Exhibition catalogue. Albury, NSW, Australia: Occupational Therapy Programme, Charles Sturt University, 2001.

Mahdi LC, Foster S, Little M (eds). Betwixt and Between: Patterns of Masculine and Feminine Initiation. La Salle, IL: Open Court, 1987.

Marsden S. Healthy Arts – A Guide to the Role of Arts in Health Care. Melbourne, Victoria, Australia: Arts Access, 1993.

Marsden S, Thiele M. Risking Art: Art for Survival. Richmond, Victoria, Australia: Jesuit Social Services, 2000.

Miller V. Necta: Not Only Fun and Games – A Study of Various Aspects of Network for Exploring Creativity in Therapy and the Arts. Unpublished Masters of Arts manuscript. Macquarie University at Sydney, NSW, Australia, 1992.

Miller V, Fox J. Creativity: The Forgotten Link in Occupational Therapy. Paper presented at the Australian Association of Occupational Therapists, 15th Federal Conference National Perspectives, Sydney, NSW, Australia, 1988.

Noonan C. Stepping Out (video recording). Sydney, Australia: Binnaburra Film Company, 1980.

Opperman M, Dreyfus E. Art, Architecture and Medicine: Place Making in Liverpool Hospital. Paper presented at the Intersections Conference, August, University of NSW, Australia, 1996.

Peppard J, Hill M, Ness B. Youth participation in health services: practical issues at the second story. In: Bennett DL, Williams M (eds), New Universals: Adolescent Health in a Time of Change. Sydney, Australia: Australian Association for Adolescent Health, 1988.

Silverstein S. The adolescent waiting room. Social Work 1973; November: 105–7.

Tindale RS, Heath L, Edwards J, Posavac EJ, Bryant FB, Suarez-Balkazar Y et al. (eds), Theory and Research on Small Groups. New York, NY: Plenum Press, 1988.

Vandenberg B, Kielhofner G. Play in evolution, culture, and individual adaptation: implications for therapy. American Journal of Occupational Therapy 1982; 36: 20–8.

VicHealth. Creative Connections for Health: Events Calendar [poster]. Melbourne, Victoria, Australia: VicHealth – Arts for Health, 2003.

Yalom ID. The Theory and Practice of Group Psychotherapy. New York, NY: Basic Books, 1975.

Yeats M. Art for art's sake: a participant observation study of artsenta. Occupation 1993; 1: 18–31.

CHAPTER 9

Group projects: experiences and outcomes of creativity

COMPILED AND EDITED BY THERESE SCHMID

> The company of others and the enjoyment of creating something is import-
> ant to well-being. (Participant comment, 'Material Women: Weaving Fabric
> and Stories')

Introduction

This chapter is a collection of writings gathered from people who have
designed and facilitated group projects in creative activities, including
arts, in various community and healthcare settings. This assemblage is not
intended to be formal research; however, it is assumed that useful consensual truth can be derived from the collection. The purpose of the
chapter is to introduce contributions from a variety of current community
groups, projects and programmes, funded by both government and non-
government organizations in order to stimulate readers to perceive
opportunities for research.

The idea for this chapter was driven by my belief that creative activities
contribute to health and well-being, and by my belief that doing creative
activities in a group situation is doubly effective for participants' health and
well-being. I have had many years of experience in co-ordinating group
psychotherapy in a therapeutic community, and in designing and leading
expressive arts groupwork sessions in adult and tertiary education, and in
health-professional settings. I have used creative arts activities to facilitate
teambuilding (recent examples include the Newcastle Family Support
Service and the Hunter Mental Health Services, NSW, Australia) and in facilitating participants' personal and social growth. However, experience is
not enough. Research is needed to examine the possible connection
between health and well-being, creative activities and groupwork.

When searching for contributions for this chapter, I was directed to
many groups and individuals through local government community and
cultural development officers, and various health and arts professionals.

All of the group projects suggested had similar objectives, which were the health and well-being of the individual and the community. I was aware that groups are often talking about the same things but have different ways of describing creativity, response feelings and health and well-being. As there were so many groups and projects offering a variety of creative activities to a variety of people, I limited the search to a cross-section of types of group. For example, it became clear, through contacts with VicServ in Victoria, Australia, that there are many funded psychosocial– psychiatric, rehabilitation services (J. Gray, personal communication, September 2003). As a result, I decided to invite two long-standing, innovative groups, 'Sound Minds' (from the UK) and 'Artsenta' (from New Zealand) to contribute. It was anticipated that their respective contributions could be excellent examples of best practice for those groups offering opportunities for people with an enduring mental illness. Both have similar philosophies; however, they are not therapy programmes. The business management field was not solicited for contributions. A wealth of literature exists on creativity in management, often referred to as innovation or invention; however, the literature shows no apparent link between such creativity and health and well-being. I was unable to gain contributions from indigenous groups. This was due to time restrictions. However, I was able to make contact with indigenous Australians in the Albury-Wodonga area of New South Wales, Australia. One woman, Rita Wenberg, agreed to write about her experience, and her contribution appears in Chapter Seven. 'Material Women: Weaving Fabric and Stories' serves as an exemplary model of design and research that could be utilized by the myriad of interesting contemporary arts and crafts groups and guilds.

I made contact with suggested groups and projects, and those that were already known to me by sending them an information letter and an invitation to write an account. The project leaders of each group were invited to describe their projects and participant outcomes. Contributions could include accounts of either 'healthy' people or of people who had 'ill-health' or 'disability'. The outcomes that I was interested in were feelings of pleasure, joy, excitement, confidence, satisfaction, self-esteem, feelings of connectedness, belonging or any other feelings (as described as sources of 'health' and 'well-being' in Chapter 1), and whether these feelings contributed to participants' health and well-being. It was also suggested that they might have examples of how people have changed their feelings and attitudes to their daily life and everyday activities as a result of gaining a positive sense of health and well-being. The project leaders were asked to describe the creative activity from which these feelings arose and to identify evaluation methods they used.

All the responses received have been included here, and nearly all of the requests for accounts received a response. Apart from minor corrections, most of the accounts are presented as they were originally written; however, a few have been edited to fit the available space. I do not attempt to analyse or interpret them. The contributions speak for themselves, and it is left to the reader to recognize how participants' responses could be the subject of useful research. Additional references and information are included at the end of some contributions with the aim of furthering opportunities for research.

The following 10 groups and projects have been included:

* The Performing Older Women's Circus and the Older People's Circus.
* Small Towns Big Picture: the art of engagement.
* Sound Minds.
* Bellbird Garden.
* Artsenta: Sunflowers, butterflies and a big, big cookie jar.
* The Inside Outside People and Magic Kingdom.
* The Wilderness Theatre Project.
* Sculpture Trail: ARTnode.
* Material Women: weaving fabric and stories.
* Development of Creativity.

The Performing Older Women's Circus

On tour in Victoria, Australia, March, 2003

Therese Schmid

The Performing Older Women's Circus (POW) was on tour in Victoria, Australia during March 2003. The ages of the women ranged between 40 and 71 years. POW was established in 1995 at the Footscray Community Arts Centre and is funded by VicHealth, a state-government-funded health-promotional initiative. The group was developed by members of the Women's Circus with the aim of creating a safe and supportive environment where older women could meet and participate in physical activity.

The Upper Hume Health Promotion Group invited POW to the region as a high-profile event promoting participation in healthy activity. It was also seen to challenge limiting beliefs about the potential and ability of older people. It aimed to show the community that older people, given the right support and training, could achieve a high level of fitness and express this in a creative and poignant way to the broader community.

I interviewed the 15 performers in a group, questioning them about their participation in the circus, their motivation and the benefits they obtained from their participation, and asked them about whether their involvement in circus, as a creative activity, benefited their health and well-being. I took notes recording the performers' comments. Performers' comments are included below. Chapter Seven also includes first-hand accounts by two performers.

Responses

All the performers agreed that the changes in their posture were beneficial and that they had increased flexibility, co-ordination and strength. They said:

'There is an emphasis on the whole body well-being, not just on the physical.'

'I am feeling a lot better about myself.'

'The group members support each other through new challenges.'

'Part of the beauty in this is that there is no competition, that there is a sense of community, each of us being supported by others in achieving our own goals.' All the women agreed to this (all nodded).

'We, as individuals, are evolving all the time; we research as a team. Acrobalances lifts our creativity with a trainer. We increase our confidence.'

'It is such a buzz and [that feeling] helps you keep going back for that buzz.'

'It is a joy in seeing other people achieving . . .'

'Through others' creativity we open up our own creativity.'

'Circus helps you relax in your life . . . being more relaxed at work and in being with the group.'

'My mind is more active in Circus. I have increased physical fitness and achieving the outcome is wonderful. There is an increase in confidence; and there is a strong sense of ownership.' (POW runs as a collective.)

Reference

Performing Older Women's Circus. Home page, 2002. (Accessed 22 March 2004: www.vicnet.net.au/~powcirc/about.htm)

The Older People's Circus Project: Fruit Bats 2003
Upper Hume Community Health Team, Wodonga, NSW, Australia

Therese Schmid

As a result of the huge response to the POW performances, the Upper Hume Community Health Team gained funding for an Older People's Circus. It was a prototype for Australia. The town of Albury houses the

National Flying Fruit Fly Circus School, and hence there was the potential for working collaboratively with the Fruit Fly Circus and their trainers to develop an Older People's Circus. At the end of a 10-week programme, two public performances were held.

The Upper Murray Community Health Centre implemented a pre- and post-evaluation that identified that the circus training and the performances had successfully facilitated participants' health and well-being. I arranged a meeting with the staff to discuss the perceived benefits to participants' health and well-being. The following is the outcome of the discussion with staff members (P. Mobach and L. Catlow, personal communication, November 27, 2003).

The staff related that the feedback gained from the participants was unanimously positive, with 100% commitment to continuing the project. Staff reported that all participants mentioned they had improved flexibility, fitness and strength; that some participants reported a loss of weight; that there was an overall sense of joy and fun about participating; that many participants mentioned overcoming physical and mental hurdles and the huge sense of accomplishment this gave them; that it gave them a feeling of confidence; that they felt happier; that they liked being more social; that they were able to laugh at themselves. Many declared that they experienced improved self-esteem and self-confidence and a general sense of well-being.

The staff discussed the rationale of health promotion through circus activity. The main purpose of circus work was that it challenged ageism and redundant beliefs about physical activity. The following comments by staff are about why the circus activity worked:

> Circus gave people experience to learn something new about themselves. It touches a childlike part of people. That is what I saw – people being young again . . . playing and having fun.

> . . . it is already about stereotype . . . All duty of care gets in the road . . . [here she was talking about the staff in community health, when staff become too preoccupied with 'duty of care' and their attitudes to ageing are stereotypical]. Circus broke this down . . . Circus was about challenging ageism and redundant beliefs. It was changing through action. This is the difference, doing an activity.

The participants and the circus trainers completed a post-evaluation questionnaire. Permission to use this material was kindly granted by the Upper Hume Community Health Team. Participants' responses to the question, 'What is the single most important thing you have gained from this project?', included:

> 'Knowing I can do things I never thought I could. And the ability to laugh at myself.'

'A greater sense of well-being, physical and mental and emotional.'

'It has been great to be with happy people and work in an encouraging and supportive environment and experience the thrill for achieving skills I thought were left behind with childhood.'

'A person is never too old to try something new.'

'Increased confidence in myself about physical and mental boundaries.'

'A huge sense of achievement.'

'The feeling that there is still a lot of life in these old bones and that I can do more than I thought.'

'Knowledge that I can do stuff I never believed I could.'

One circus trainer commented that the team felt excited to see 'people grow in confidence' as they learnt new skills and met challenges as they arose. The trainers are strongly committed to continuing their involvement in the project.

Following the enormous success of the project, Upper Hume Community Health has agreed to fund a further 10-week programme to maintain the energy, fitness and skill level acquired. Interest has been high, with all 40 places filled. Negotiations are under way to develop the Older People's Circus as an ongoing project.

References and resources

Women's Circus and the Older Women's Circus. Home page, 2003. (Accessed 22 March 2003: www.vicnet.au/~powcirc/about.htm)
VicHealth. Creative Connections: Promoting Mental Health and Well-being through Community Arts Participation. Melbourne, Victoria, Australia: Victoria Health Promotion Foundation, 2002.

'The Young at Heart chorus' is an arts project that aims to break down ageism beliefs about health and well-being. This was presented at the Melbourne International Arts Festival (Victoria, Australia) in October, 2003. The average age of the performers was 80 years.

'Heartsongs', a funded creative project, was aimed to assist the mental well-being of participants with cancer. The project consisted of workshops which encouraged participants to write 'from the heart' in exploring their emotions and experiences of breast cancer. This project was a current-affairs item on Stateline Victoria on 24 October, 2003. (Accessed 25 October, 2003: www.abc.net.au/stateline/vic/content/2003/ s974741.htm)

Small Towns Big Picture: the art of engagement

Victoria, Australia

Judy Spokes, Cultural Development Network

'Small Towns Big Picture' was an innovative regional development project of the Cultural Development Network of Victoria and the Centre for Sustainable Regional Communities at La Trobe University in Bendigo, Victoria. It involved the active and creative engagement of the towns-people of five small towns in central Victoria and was supported by their respective shires.

Small Towns Big Picture used a mix of creative processes led by community-based artists and the Cultural Development Network, and research and community planning techniques led by the university. Its purpose was to develop a clear understanding (or benchmark) of each town's current performance relative to long-term indicators of sustainability (economic, environmental and social). The project's objective was to focus and stimulate future action plans to tackle sustainability at the local level.

It was the inclusion of commissioned artists and a cultural-development approach that achieved the project's critical goal of actively engaging townspeople in the social research and community-planning exercise which, otherwise, might have been regarded as dull, unimportant or relevant only to town élites (Hawkes, 2001). It was also the arts approach that catalysed community interest and vitality, and enabled the project to be further developed locally to create and build on other community-building initiatives. A key goal was to model a broader and more embedded role for the arts in community-capacity-building programmes in regional areas, and to highlight – especially for local government – the powerful potential of creative strategies for community engagement.

The first phase of the project concluded on 25 October, 2002 and exceeded all partners' best expectations. The arts results of the project include the following.

* The creation and presentation (in each town) of a musical play, 'Right Where We Are'. This reflected on life from the different points of view of the participating towns (ideas sourced through a series of focus groups). The play was performed by townspeople and featured original music and songs composed by Craig Christie. It was acclaimed by standing ovations and encores in every town. The town halls were packed to standing room only – almost unprecedented in many towns.
* A CD soundtrack of the songs of the musical production (significant commercial potential exists for some of these).

- A concert featuring approximately a dozen local amateur and professional performances in each town made up the first half of the Small Towns Big Picture event and was followed after intermission by the original play.
- Schoolchildren and others in the five towns enjoyed a series of art-making workshops exploring the project themes (e.g. ecological footprint analyses). These resulted in the exhibition, at each Small Towns Big Picture event, of a beautiful collection of art works (ceramics, printmaking, pin-hole photography and banners) that decorated the town hall venues and streets, and featured in information and research displays prepared by the university. Community artist Andrea Hicks co-ordinated this component of the project with other local artists. The works were subsequently exhibited at the City Gallery in Melbourne's CBD in April–June 2003.
- An interactive website that documents the connections within groups and agencies in each town (and also identifies gaps). Designed by local artist, Anne Moloney, the website will be further developed by participating towns and will continue to grow.
- Film-maker Phillip Ashton has documented the results of the project (and processes leading up to them) in his film, 'A Journey in Community Building'. The film demonstrates the value of the project to artists, councils, communities and regional development authorities.

Small Towns Big Picture is a useful new model for future practice and will be of interest to anyone concerned with new and creative ways to strengthen communities towards sustainability. Further resources are available on the following web pages:

- www.smalltownsbigpicture.com.au (for further information on Small Towns Big Picture; accessed 5 June 2004).
- www.ccd.net (for information on the Community Development Network).
- www.thehumanities.com (for information on humanities in general).

Reference

Hawkes J. Fourth Pillar of Sustainability: Culture's Essential Role in Public Planning. Victoria, Australia: Cultural Development Network and Common Ground Publishing, 2001.

Further information

'The Torch Project' facilitates 'Re-Igniting Community' by providing a platform in a non-threatening public forum for marginalized communities and individuals who have little opportunity to express their needs and desires. It is a Community Cultural Development initiative. It has been supported by 200-plus indigenous, government, church, educational, business and community organizations, contributing approximately $600,000 as at February 2003. Local social issues and related community needs are identified and given voice in the context of the history of the community. These issues are addressed in an ongoing process, via community consultation, workshops, activities in schools, theatrical and artistic expression, and ongoing community-development activities driven by the local communities. The team has been able to identify and demonstrate community need, and clearly link this need with the outcomes delivered. The University of Technology, Sydney's Centre for Popular Education, is currently compiling findings from an in-depth evaluation and analysis of the project's community building achievements, in order to examine the individual and community impact of the project. (Accessed 8 October, 2003: www.thetorch.asn.au).

The Centre for Popular Education, University of Technology, Sydney, Australia. The Centre studies and supports popular educational practice which serves the interests of people who are marginalized, and are engaged in advocacy, social action or community development activities. Members of the Centre research and teach in a range of arenas including schools, health promotion, youth work or education, international and community development, adult and community education, basic education, social movements and unions. The topics include the arts and social change, creative capacity building, education and social action. (Accessed 16 May, 2004: www.cpe.uts.edu.au).

Sound Minds

Battersea, South West London, UK

Paul Brewer

Sound Minds (www.soundminds.co.uk) is a small independent registered charity and company limited by guarantee. It provides opportunities for people with enduring mental health problems to be involved in music and other arts activities.

History

Sound Minds was founded in 1994 by an occupational therapist and a group of service users. It was initially supported financially and managerially by the Methodist Church, which owns the basement studio. The service users had spent much of their lives within the mental health system in a devalued patient role. They were demanding 'art for art's sake' rather than art in the furtherance of therapy. The Sound Minds ethos is, therefore, one of empowerment and social inclusion through the arts. The majority of the management committee and staff team are artists and musicians who experience mental health problems. Most originally came to receive the service they now help to provide. Some came with pre-existing skills in the arts, as actors, painters, musicians and designers, and were able to share these skills with others, to the benefit of the project.

Membership

All Sound Minds members are referred by community mental health teams and remain under their care. The project engages a high proportion of service users estranged from mainstream services, including people from black and minority ethnic backgrounds (41% of the membership). On average, 40–50 people per week use the facilities in Battersea, and we have about 50 active members. In 2002–2003, 90% of members have received a psychotic diagnosis (bipolar affective disorder or a schizophrenic illness).

'Sound Advice'

The national significance of the work of Sound Minds with black and minority ethnic groups was recognized by the Department of Health in 2000. The Department awarded a three-year grant to the charity to develop 'Sound Advice'. This was to be a national project advising organizations in the field on practical aspects of applying the arts in mental health, and user empowerment. A team of service users now gives regular talks, workshops and performances throughout the UK, and Sound Minds successfully hosted its own conference in 2003 on the arts in mental health.

Fighting stigma

Achievements in the arts erode negative stereotypes of mental ill health in the public mind. Our regular music and poetry performances and drama and visual art events are a strong focus for news stories, opening the channels of communication to the general population and raising awareness of mental health issues. Consequently, Sound Minds has received disproportionate attention from national television and radio. A group of our members have undergone media training and are now comfortable about sharing their experiences of mental ill-health with journalists. They are committed to making best use of these opportunities to challenge stigma as it arises.

Social inclusion

Sound Minds recognizes the social exclusion suffered by people with severe and enduring mental-health problems. They suffer the primary impact of mental ill-health on functioning and the consequences for social networks, employment and advancement. Sound Minds is committed to overcoming this impact through: the provision of flexible training with assistance from adult education skilled and experienced support, professionally delivered by staff, volunteers and other service users; a focus on personal creativity; an ethos of mutual respect and co-operation, user empowerment and enablement; arts initiatives with a primary or secondary aim of challenging stigma; embedding Sound Minds in the local community.

Sound Minds is an active partner in 'Healthy Living in Battersea', a coalition of health-related organizations. Sound Minds is represented at board level by two of our service users. It is working towards membership of the London Open College Network.

Weekly sessions currently include:

- Live music: the live-music studio is equipped with a PA system, drums, keyboards, backline and effects. Members of these sessions have formed bands, and most are performing. The bands include: 'The Atlantans' (pop standards of the 1960s and 1970s), 'Turquoise Blue' (pop and reggae standards from the 1960s to the 1980s), 'The Moodcutters' (dark indie pop), 'Mean Machine' (rock), 'Mumbo Jumbo' (blues), 'Bluesology' (blues), 'Channel One' (reggae) and 'Devil's Bones' (rock).
- Music technology: there are seven sessions throughout the week, some individual, some in small groups. The sessions include a range of popular music styles, using two PCs with programs such as 'Cubase', 'Sonar' and 'Reason', a mixer, sound modules, keyboards and effects.
- Visual art: the 'depARTmental' art studio is open for staffed sessions twice per week. It is staffed by visual artists who are mental-health-service users and have teaching qualifications. The majority of artists are painters.
- Web design: there are ad hoc individual sessions using Microsoft 'Frontpage' and Adobe 'Photoshop'.
- Creative writing: the group 'basemental' meets weekly for all aspects of the written word (poetry, lyric writing), also incorporating music technology to develop musical settings.
- Drama: the 'Theatre of Visions' has weekly workshops, leading to occasional performances such as 'The Anansi Web Show' at the Battersea Arts Centre in 2000.
- Video-making: there is one regular staffed session, plus ad hoc work throughout the week, producing music videos, pop promos, videos of live performances and mental health promotion work (aspects of mental-health service-user experiences).

Evidence of the positive impact of arts activities on mental health

An independent undergraduate qualitative study at Sound Minds, (Merrick, 2003), yielded the following:

> 'I've struck up a friendship with a bass player. Now, me being a drummer, you're meant to strike up a good relationship with the bass player, but we've taken it a stage further where we go down the pub every time we meet.'

> '. . . we get on together, because we've got something similar. And if you're performing, doing things together, that helps a lot you know.'

One participant described how a successful performance enhances self-esteem:

> 'When they do applaud and say, "Yeah, that's good," it makes me think that I've done something that they can't take something away from. And that gives me a bit of a lift. I feel more positive about myself, that I'm not useless.'

A second evaluation took place in February 2003. A questionnaire was evolved with the help of a researcher attached to a group of local family doctors. It was based on a national measure of health outcomes for healthy living centres. Twenty-nine questionnaires were distributed and administered by a service user. Twenty-seven (59% of active membership) completed questionnaires were returned; 60% of respondents had attended Sound Minds for more than one year. The majority of respondents (88%) rated the Sound Minds service as good or excellent.

Asked what they liked most about Sound Minds, the most often-mentioned were friendships and creativity.

Friendships

The commonality of the creative interest was remarked upon, as were strong conditions for the development of friendship ties:

> 'People are friendly, supportive and with many things in common with each other.'

> 'I like the good camaraderie with other band members.'

> 'I like the fact that I can get on with everybody and have found some good people to work with.'

> 'I like the chance to play with other like-minded people/musicians.'

Creativity

Respondents welcomed the outlet for creativity:

> 'I like realizing creativity.'

'I like how you can express your artistic ideas.'

'I relax when I play music.'

In addition to the research, the following useful comment was made by one of the service users, Sonja Cooper:

'I suffer from bipolar affective disorder and I'm currently in recovery. Being creative helps to motivate me. I think partly because art is practical. Doing something inspires me to do more in other areas of my life – to go places and see things. When I'm actually creating something I feel positive, I feel energized. I also find it very calming, it helps to alleviate any anxiety I may be feeling. I just can't imagine a life without art and the opportunity to be creative.'

Mental health outcomes

Respondents were also asked what difference Sound Minds had made to their lives, by indicating how much they agreed or disagreed with a set of statements. The statements were generated by a focus group of users, and some were taken from a health evaluation questionnaire commissioned by the Department of Health:

Outcome (%)

More of a sense of purpose (81)

More friends (78)

Felt happier (77)

Felt more confident (76).

Reference

Merrick I. How clients with long-term mental health problems use a community based music project to create therapeutic social networks. Mental Health Occupational Therapy 2003; 8: July.

Additional references and resources

Established arts based services like 'The Artful Dodgers Studio', Richmond, Victoria, Australia, use arts for 'recovery' as opposed to 'therapy' (Marsden and Thiele, 2002; Thiele and Marsden, 2003). These services provide those with a mental illness with a community, participant-based arts-studios approach (Pepper, 2003). The creative activity, whether music or art, seems to be chosen by the participant as a vehicle for recovery, for skill building, and for self-expression. Creative activities are often described as providing opportunities for self-expression, personal growth and improving well-being (Rubbins, 1987; Yeats, 1993).

Many non-Government services in Victoria provide various models of arts-based services for people with a mental illness. Refer to Psychiatric Disability Services of Victoria (VICSERV) Inc. Australia, and www.vicserv.org.au (accessed 5 June, 2004) and the VICSERVE journal, *New Paradigm. The Australian Journal on Psychosocial Rehabilitation*.

Jackson C. Making music. Mental Health Care 1999, 21, 348–349.
Jackson C. Music, meaning and mental health. Occupational Therapy News 2000, October, 24.
Marsden S, Thiele M. (ed.). Risking Art. Art for Survival. Outlining the Role of the Arts in Services to Marginalised Young People. Richmond: Jesuit Social Services, 2002.
Neami Splash Art Studio Evaluation. The secret life of splash. Putting words to a visual experience. Preston, Victoria, Australia: Neami Splash Art Studio, 2003.
Pepper S. Arts-based practice in psychosocial rehabilitation. New Paradigm. The Australian Journal of Psychosocial Rehabilitation 2003; 1: 46–53.
Rubbins JA. Art Therapy Approaches. Theory and Technique. New York, NY: Brunner/Mazel, 1987.
Scrogings, Z. YPPI Creative Arts Project 1998–1999. Children and Young People's Prevention and Early Intervention Centre. Central Coast Health, NSW, Australia: YPPI Centre 1999.
Thiele M, Marsden S. Engaging Art. The Artful Dodgers Studio. A Theoretical Model of Practice. Richmond, Victoria, Australia: Jesuit Social Services, 2003.
Yeats M. Arts for arts sake. A participant observation study of Artsenta. Occupation 1993; 1: 18–31.

Bellbird Garden

Morisset Hospital, Hunter Valley Health Services, NSW, Australia

Justin Steele

'Bellbird Garden' is a pre-vocational training programme based in horti-culture. It is part of the Psychiatric Rehabilitation Services at Morisset Hospital, for the Hunter Mental Health Service, NSW. It services a range of clients with mental illness from both the hospital and the community. It consists of a certified organic market garden and a small wholesale nur-sery and operates from Monday to Friday, staffed by an occupational therapist and a vocational instructor.

The core philosophy of the garden is based on encouraging individual strengths, experiential learning and hands-on participation. It is about matching clients with a suitable task, no matter how small, in order to con-tribute to the overall group task. For example, in a creative exercise for a client who is restless and unable to concentrate during a mosaic activity, the client could instead be used to break up the tiles, which is a more physical and a less mentally taxing activity than placing the tiles in the correct pattern.

Art has played an increasing role in the programme over the years. It started with a gifted client who was an arts graduate. The garden was his canvas. Our tunnel house provided him with a studio. Each day he would attend the garden and paint. We ended up with an array of totem poles, a mural on our tool shed, and corrugated iron sheets used as canvases for his distinctive style, inspired by Aboriginal dot painting.

Since then we have embraced outdoor art as an essential part of our programme. We have mosaic bed-number markers, decorative plant supports, brightly painted bird boxes, totem poles, giant insects made from wood, wire and mosaic, a giant, wire spider's web decorated with coloured, tumbled glass, a carved, hebel-stone water-feature and gumboot planters. Some of the sculptures are practical, some just decorative. We see that the predominantly male population has responded well to the large scale of the projects and the woodwork, metalwork and tiling aspects of the tasks.

It has also been a way of engaging people on another level, to introduce them to another side of gardening, provide diversity in activities that we offer and provide an element of exploration and fun.

Most of our projects have involved minimal costs, as we have utilized recycled materials such as donated tiles, salvaged timber or common everyday objects that have been discarded.

This year also saw us enter a sculpture competition called 'Waste as Art'. With a theme of recycling and supported by a local government sponsorship, it was exhibited at the Newcastle Regional Museum. Our entry was 'Songbirds', and was based on recycled aluminium cans fashioned into birds that were sitting on an old fence in the arrangement of a musical score. For this we took the $1000 first prize in our division. The highlights of the process were in attending the public opening of the exhibition with the clients who participated in its creation, and in one of them getting up to accept the prize on the group's behalf. Another client said, on the night, that he guessed that this made the group a bit of a role model for others. It had seen them go from being 'just patients' to being there on the night as exhibitors and prizewinners, proving that anyone could give it a go.

We have just received word that Rotary and the Lions Club are giving us $3000 towards our sculpture garden. This will help us to create a separate sculpture garden in the grounds of the hospital for all to use and enjoy. This will be a blend of art and landscaping, and will incorporate seating areas for the clients to enjoy with other hospital residents, and for their families to enjoy during visits. The sculpture garden will feature works produced by the clients in a variety of mediums. They will reflect the bushland surrounds as well as aspects of hospital life, based on themes such as friendship, understanding, family and acceptance.

So, gardening and creativity are not mutually exclusive activities. Our garden and nursery are filled with examples that help to create an overall atmosphere for the programme. It shows that the Bellbird programme is not a sterile or purely clinical environment. It is, instead, promoting and accepting of individual differences and individual contributions. The art that surrounds us helps to identify us as unique. It offers a more holistic view of what the hospital is all about, and that is the individual.

Artsenta: Sunflowers, butterflies and a big, big cookie jar

Artsenta participants, Dunedin, New Zealand

The following extracts from the life and work of its artists and support folk illustrate the values of being involved in 'Artsenta'.

Artsenta (www.artsenta.cjb.net) is a community art workshop. It is a non-therapeutic, supportive community in which personal creativity and expression are encouraged to develop and flourish. It is funded by the Departments of Health, of Work and Income, and charitable trusts, and is also supported by local businesses. The Creative Arts Trust set up Artsenta 18 years ago and its mission is to provide opportunities for artists in the mental-health community to work in the arts.

As we go up the stairs into our Artsenta studio space, there are murals on either side of us. There are also rules so our space will be as safe as we can make it – for ourselves and for everyone else.

If you called in one day you might find a lot of people here, or only a few. There may be only a few of us because of what is going on inside or outside the studio itself. (We may be visiting a member's exhibition at a local venue, or visiting a local stone quarry together.) And for the same reason you may find the place bursting at the doors (there may be a public exhibition in our own gallery, or a poetry evening).

Around us at the moment, inside, are new lives arising from a piano – very creative works are appearing from every part of it every day, and as they are created, there may well be a musical accompaniment coming from the other piano at the same time.

There are still copies of the Newsletter and the photos of the end of the 2003 'Alexandra Blossom Festival' where many of us went (to share appearing as sunflowers with our colleagues from Clyde!). And in the middle of all this there is the book, *The Song of the Belly Button Man*, to keep looking at, and relooking at, and showing to visitors, and recalling for them – and ourselves – its launch at the Dunedin Railway Station Gallery – along with all the local poets who had put words with the works of the Artsenta artists. In it, some of the artists said about their own creative experience in this beautifully presented book:

'I'm enjoying coming to the Artsenta and I love working on my artwork – it's what keeps me going.' (E.G. Peach)

'I like to paint flowers and butterflies, and to use bright colours. The butterflies remind me of a free spirit.' (N.C.)

And right here, in the middle of all this and alongside the others, in his corner of the space, Kevin Dewe works on his 'Big, Big Cookie Jar'. Kevin is a prolific craftsperson and stops to say a few words about what he is doing (which he is always very willing to do), and what it is to be a member of the Artsenta community:

> What I am making at the moment is a cookie jar. A big, big cookie jar like a strawberry. It's cooking at the moment, and I hope to paint it next week . . . I get a lot of ideas for my art work, I think about it a lot, about the things I like to make. I make a lot here and a lot at home. It is good that you have someone to help you. I have miles of things I've done here – a dog for Heather Martin, big, big fish . . .

Kevin brings mountains of creativity with him each time he arrives through the doors. But he knows well (as do we all who contribute in all our different roles) and appreciates the integrity, which includes the materials, the space, the patient teaching and sharing of expertise. It also includes support and tolerance, management and administration, and the persistence of liaison, policy-writing and fund-raising, which for 18 years has remained true to the vision – that the creativity of art is not only the birthright of humankind, it is humankind, no matter what. And that means the total commitment to that vision of every one of us, inside and out, no matter how hard this can sometimes get, because creativity is not just freedom and personal expression. It is the freedom to be responsible for what we create.

We have always had that clear vision. And absolute integrity. For 18 years. Through thick and thin, staff changes and space changes and Government changes. Perhaps that's one of the reasons we're still around. And the evidence? The evidence is in the art.

Additional resources and information

www.artsenta.cjb.net (retrieved June 5, 2004)

Caulton RF (ed.). The Best of Occupation, 1993–2003. Dunedin, NZ: School of Occupational Therapy, Otago Polytechnic, 2003.

West R. The Song of the Belly Button Man: A Meeting of Art and Poetry. Dunedin, NZ: Artsenta, 2002.

The Inside Outside People, the Magic Kingdom and other projects

Developed by John Hunter Hospital Arts for Health for Children's Hospital, Newcastle, NSW, Australia; co-ordinated by Pippa Robinson; artist, Belinda Russell

Pippa Robinson

I first met Belinda Russell in 2001 when she submitted her paintings and drawings to the John Hunter Hospital, Arts for Health, for exhibition. Her successful exhibition, 'The Land of Creative Freedom', which delighted the hospital community, led to Belinda becoming a volunteer, both with the hospital's 'Play Programme' and for a project with Arts for Health – the creation of the 'Inside Outside People'.

The Inside Outside People

Belinda Russell and Denise Yabsley (a Play Programme volunteer) met young people on the wards and persuaded those who were willing to lie down on paper on the ground and have their body outline traced. The children giggled and laughed, but kept still enough for the tracings. These were then transferred onto board and cut out ready to be painted. The images became generic as many children helped to paint the Inside Outside People. One patient, however, took special delight in creating her very own character.

The Inside Outside People project was developed to involve children who, because of illness, spend much of their time in hospital. These young, sick people experience a life in hospital that is quite different to their ordinary life at home. It was suggested to them that they paint different aspects of their lives on each side of the cut-outs: hospital life on one side and outside life on the other. They had intense discussions about the effect of hospitalization on their young lives and the things that they missed most from life outside.

The Inside Outside People then developed their own lives as the children determined the characters of their cut-out people. Several children worked together on one piece, and families, staff and visitors picked up paintbrushes too. People became absorbed in the fun of painting and deciding what colour and what embellishment to add next. Each person added their own individual mark to the work, taking great pride in their contribution.

One young patient decided to portray dancing and having fun at home and school on one side. On her hospital side, against a green background, which referred to her illness, she pasted photos of her treatments and hospital carers and friends. She carefully added real tubing to her cut-out nose to create the oxygen lines she so often had to wear when ill in hospital.

The aim was to allow the participants to be in control of the work. When in hospital, patients lose control of many events and procedures, even the environment, and they can feel disempowered. This was a project to empower. The children had choices to make and painting to do. The emphasis at the time was on the process of making, not on the end result.

The Inside Outside People responded to the different needs of the participants. As the characters of the cut-outs developed, so the children found satisfaction. For some the activity was entertaining. They were able to ignore the hospital world as they worked together having fun. Others thought more seriously about their life in hospital and enjoyed expressing their feelings in developing their 'person'.

Once the characters were complete, the cut-out children took off, visiting various spots in the corridors of the hospital, before spending time enlivening the entrance to hide the renovations for the new Emergency Department. Here, the children and Belinda added their own flower garden, which they painted on the hoardings behind the cut-outs. Security staff added dark glasses and a cap to the cut-out of a young man with a broken arm. When Belinda had her back turned, one young boy, a talented artist, painted an enormous Venus Fly Trap plant hovering over a small girl waving a bunch of flowers. He wore an artist's beret, and amused the staff on the information counter opposite with his antics. The delight and admiration of people walking through the main entrance of the hospital greatly boosted the self-esteem of this normally quiet boy.

The Magic Kingdom

Belinda Russell, having established a rapport with some of the children, was then commissioned to work at John Hunter Hospital with young people who were suffering with cystic fibrosis. The patients had requested a new look for the isolation room where they had to stay when in hospital. Together, they decided to create the Magic Kingdom. As leading magician, Belinda created a warm, safe haven full of laughter, design, paintings and fun. With help from the children, the room was transformed into the Magic Kingdom. This room-in-the-making was much loved by staff, patients, families and all who visited the ward and entered the magical room.

The Magic Kingdom gave so much pleasure, especially to two young people in their last few months of life. The planning, painting and fun was a distraction from the hard reality of illness for the patients, their families and staff. The opening of the room was a very special and happy day. Everyone dressed up, and one of the children spoke eloquently of the importance of the project and of the sponsors who had helped make their dream a reality. It was a great party.

The success of the Magic Kingdom led to the sponsorship of another artwork, which the children requested for the physiotherapy department. This area, where they had to spend much time, was also frequented by adult patients, and was a dull, curtained area at the end of the department. It became 'Circus Carnivale', with bright tumblers and jugglers looking down on the exercise and treatment area. A second isolation room was also sponsored and this became 'The Secret Garden'. Belinda has developed interactive books for these children to use while they stay in the Magic Kingdom and the Secret Garden.

The projects continue to help with healing, particularly for the young patients who use the rooms. I remember meeting the first patient in the Secret Garden. She pointed out, with joy, the elf she had just found hiding by the bed and flying a kite. However, there are also the happy memories of the creation of the artworks, which provide some comfort to the grieving families who have lost a child.

Matthew (artist, aged 8 years), talking about his cut-out:

'The mouth is like that because he's happy and scared. He's scared because someone might take him away. He wants his sword.'

Kimberly (artist, aged 16 years):

'The arts are really great because I don't sit around feeling sorry for myself, or thinking about being sick, because I've got something to make. I didn't really know what art was really for until I made my cut-out. There should be more art people at the hospital and a place especially to do art.'

Belinda Russell (artist co-ordinator):

'As one of the artists in residence at the John Hunter Children's Hospital, I have had the privilege to be involved with some wonderful people and projects. It has been so rewarding to see the benefits that art and creativity bring to hospitalized children, their families and staff. I have shared in the beauty and honesty that comes from the creative expression and enthusiasm of young people, and the excitement of transforming the environment around them with their help. It has been a remarkable learning experience and a unique challenge for me to work within the confines of the hospital environment, responding to the needs of each child. It was great to see the growth and sense of achievement that the children experienced as they overcame obstacles, acquired new skills and discovered talents they never realized they had. I feel honoured to have been welcomed into the hospital community and to see my art make it a more colourful and magical place to be.

I will always be grateful that I have worked on these projects. They have been very special experiences for me, both as an artist and as a human being.

Sponsors for these projects

Tilligerry Lions Club, Chroma Australia Pty Ltd, The Paint Works, Margaret Harris, The Church of the Good Shepherd Craft Group, John Hunter Children's Hospital Kids Club, Newcastle Permanent Building Society and Kimberly.

Further resources

Eames P. The Art and Health Partnership. Wellington, NZ: An Arts Access Aotearoa Publication, 1999.
Haldane D, Loppert S (eds). The Arts in Health Care. Learning from Experience. London: King's Fund Publishing in association with Lulham Art, 1999.
Kaye C, Blee T. (eds). The Arts in Health Care. A Palette of Possibilities. London: Jessica Kingsley, 1997.
The Arts for Health Research Centre, NSW, Australia. (Accessed 1 December 2003: www.placemaking.com.au)

Wilderness Theatre project

Bellingen, NSW, Australia

Kym Pitman

Art is the free continuation of the natural processes. (Goethe; as cited in Nobel, 1996, p. 101)

'The experience was indeed a peak in my overall education as it changed my entire perception of how I look at the world.' (Participant response)

'Wilderness Theatre' is an innovative methodology that uses wilderness experience to inspire and stimulate creativity, to enhance self-esteem, to develop new insights and options, and to build a voice, through theatre, by which participants express what 'really matters' to them.

As a teacher of creative arts for the Department of Education, I have found schools to be fragmented places. Yet, education in the modern world simply reflects the fragmentation of our society. I am concerned that our society suffers from overspecialization, fragmentation, co-dependency, judgementalism and technological distraction. In the wake of these, we become fragmented as humans and confused about our sense of belonging and relationship to the world. This defies our very nature as beings made up of a complex and fragile interaction of intellect, emotion, physicality and spirituality. In the face of globalization, we live in a world fraught with increasing psychotic and immune disorders, crime, conflict, and ecological, environmental and social crisis. Allen (1970) shares this concern – speaking of the need for people to awaken from:

> the lethargy of neglect and complacency of thinking induced by the present age of over-dependence on the intellect and specialization, with the accompanying heaven on earth technological developments threatening greater and greater erosion of mans [sic] humanity and his life as a true human being. (p. 17)

Having created a duality between nature and civilization where the latter feeds in devastating manner off the former, we have lost our ability to live in harmony with our environment and, particularly, our natural environment. It is through understanding and knowing oneself in relationship to the natural world around us that we develop a sense of belonging and self-confidence. The forms, proportions and creative life forces that make up the human being, we share with the rest of the natural world. Doczi (1981, p. 141) stated 'the proportions of reciprocal sharing, nature's own golden proportions, are built into our nature, into our bodies and minds which are, after all, part of nature'. It is in understanding and respecting this that our own sense of belonging can really exist. Our relationship to creation, to the natural harmony of sharing, both with each other and the environment – this is our fundamental relationship, and it is when we lose sight of this that we become lost.

If many of our youth are suffering great confusion, a sense of hopelessness, a lack of confidence about their place and role in the world, then somewhere we have lost the balance. We have fragmented our relationship with the whole, and lost our sense of harmony and sharing. The question arising here is about how to redress education in order to restore the balance, the sense of wonder, and the sense of relationship to each other and the environment. This involves two main focus areas of equal importance. The first is to address the importance of relationship with the natural environment as a basis for physical and emotional well-being. The second is to address the fragmentation of the educational process by offering holistic and meaningful creative educational experiences. Against this background, I set out to establish Wilderness Theatre as an arts-based methodology that would address both focus areas. This involved an examination of wilderness experience as a group process in terms of a creative response, with the study set in an educational context. Wilderness experience, in this process, is an extended period of time (at least a week) in a place that is unmodified by humans and isolated from civilization. It involves sleeping outdoors and covering substantial distances by foot, horse or canoe.

A group of 10 participants, aged 13–16 years, was selected for the

Bellingen Wilderness Youth Theatre Project. This eight-month, community- arts project consisted firstly of a series of preparatory workshops, followed by a wilderness trek. The insights, value clarification and perspectives gained via this wilderness experience were then explored, developed and integrated, through creative workshopping, into a piece of theatre. Participants were asked to focus on what had become important to them as a result of their wilderness experience, and this became the driving force behind the group-devised theatre workshops. The next stage was the production and public performance of the play.

Group-devised theatre involves a workshop process from which emerges a piece of theatre created by the collaborative work of a group of people. Group-devised theatre is a very effective process for creative integration of the many levels of insight and sensory, emotional and physical understanding, gained through a wilderness experience. The significance of the devising process in Wilderness Theatre is not only in enabling a group of people to articulate their views, values and opinions, but to collaboratively give voice to their freshly honed ideas and perceptions through artistic expression. The wilderness experience and the process of creating group-devised theatre have a unique relationship, in that they both address group collaboration and bonding, self-esteem, self-awareness, reflection, spontaneity, imagination, creativity, physicality, and particularly, a clarifying of perspectives and values.

The Bellingen Wilderness Youth Theatre Project was the subject of an arts-based, research enquiry incorporating a single case study. The resulting play, in the spirit of symbolic constructivism, was the analysis of stimuli arising from the wilderness experience. By utilizing enactive enquiry as researcher, I also maintained the role of participant and facilitator. The final analysis in this research was in the form of a reflective narrative based on researcher observation and participant response. It examined how the wilderness experience functions as stimulus in group-devised theatre. At the same time, it examined how the insights and awareness attained by participants in the wilderness were explored, developed, and integrated through creative processing. As a result of this, a broad range of outcomes was identified.

The emergence of the creative response, from its inception in the wilderness to its final production, gave rise to personal and social development as well as educational outcomes across curriculum frameworks. The consistent development of these outcomes infused the development of the project, as well as ultimately resulting in important long-term educational and life-related outcomes for participants. These outcomes, listed below, are not only of significant educational value in the context of learning, but also provide a sound basis for the ongoing well-being and personal happiness of participants.

The outcomes include:

* willingness to change and embrace new perspectives
* willingness and ability to question
* willingness and ability to set goals and directions
* commitment and dedication
* co-operation, collaboration and tolerance in teamwork
* intellectual rigour
* exploration of creative solutions and use of symbolism
* self-evaluation
* development of language, self-expression, and communication
* confidence and self-esteem
* knowledge and skills in integrated disciplines.

Such a project with young people provides meaningful educational experience which embodies the past and present life experiences of participants, and assists them in a constructive way in their transition into adulthood. It provides a setting in which deep human understanding can be engendered, nurtured and creatively expressed.

The combination of wilderness experience and creative integration through group-devised theatre has a profound effect upon the participants' understanding of, and compassion towards, one another, the environment and themselves. It helps to redefine values and to synthesize experiences into an understanding of what is meaningful in one's life; it provides the opportunity to let go of the extraneous and to experience freedom, spirituality and insight:

> 'The experience was indeed a peak in my overall education as it changed my entire perception of how I look at the world.' (Participant response)

References

Allen P. Education as An Art. (Rudolf Steiner and Other Writers). USA: Library of Congress, 1970.

Doczi G. The Power of Limits: Proportional Harmonies in Nature, Art and Architecture. Boulder, CO: Shambhala, 1981.

Nobel A. Educating Through Art. The Steiner School Approach. Manchester: Cromwell Press, 1996.

Additional information and resources

'Champions of Change: The Impact of the Arts on Learning' is a 1999 report which compiles seven major studies that provide new evidence of enhanced learning and achievement when students are involved in a variety of arts experiences (Accessed

14 November, 2003: www.pcah.gov). 'Champions of Change' was an American initiative, developed with the support of several organizations and the President's
Committee on the Arts and the Humanities. The studies in this report firmly conclude that learning in the arts has significant effects. Learning in that domain
supports and stimulates learning in others. Other findings reveal that learning
through the arts nurtures the development of cognitive, social, and personal com-
petencies. This is a promising lead for researchers, to design further studies
examining the possible connection with health and well-being.

'Windmill Performing Arts', Adelaide, South Australia. The company's mission is
to provide children and families with a wide range of high-quality performance
experiences that are engaging, enthralling and inspiring, and enrich children's
participation in cultural life, education and learning. Windmill works in partnership with government and non-government organizations to research and achieve
its goals. Windmill Performing Arts has an active arts education programme.
Teachers' skills, knowledge and experience are key features in the delivery of
quality arts education. Windmill is working with schools exploring issues and
policies relating to the impact of the arts on children's learning. The work focuses on aesthetic education and critical literacy. (Accessed 7 October, 2003:
www.windmill.org.au/programme.html).

White R. Public Spaces for Young People. Canberra, Australia: Australian Youth
   Foundation, National Campaign Against Violence and Crime, 1998.

Sculpture Trail: ARTnode

Newcastle, NSW, Australia

Jenny Brown, author and co-ordinator, and Cindi Hankinson

Newcastle's first accessible 'Sculpture Trail', a community arts project,
was recently completed at the University of Newcastle, NSW, Australia. It
was a large, complex piece of work, co-ordinated by Jenny Brown, which
involved 11 artists, over 100 participants, a steering committee and
numerous disability sector services. The Centenary of Federation, and
state and federal government arts agencies provided grants, with many
organizations donating materials. Marginalized community groups took
part in the project. These included people with a disability from
Newcastle and Hunter Community Access, people from the Living with
Memory Loss Group, indigenous people, and individual artists who have
a physical disability. They participated in various sculpture workshops and
horticultural practices to learn creative skills, enjoy the benefits of self-
expression and assist their groups within the wider community. Access
components were developed for the project to take into consideration
the physical and intellectual access to artworks in the environment. Four

carved sculptures and a stone slab that provides access information for the trail were created, and a CD audio guide (Brown, 2003) was developed.

A small exploratory, qualitative study was conducted with six 'Sculpture Trail: ARTnode' participants (Hankinson, unpublished). The study aimed to investigate the relationship between creativity and health with a group of people who were engaging in a community creative activity or project of their choice, rather than in a therapeutic context. Two of the participants had intellectual disabilities. One of these also had a severe physical disability. Two support workers involved with those participants and two spouses of people with memory loss were interviewed. All participants were actively involved in the creative activities.

There were three main themes identified from the data: 'Being engaged in creating', 'Creating a stronger sense of self' and 'Developing connectedness with others'. These themes indicated that creative activities provided unique experiences of absorption through creative engagement, choice through creation, and the expression of identity. In addition, they provided opportunity for connectedness with others. These experiences, in turn, enhanced the participants' sense of control, self-esteem, identity, enjoyment and motivation, as well as capacity to cope with stress, pain and negative emotions. For these participants, the results indicated a positive relationship between engaging in the creative activity and their well-being.

References

Brown J. ARTzone; environmental rehabilitation, aesthetic activism and community empowerment. Cultural geographies in practice. Cultural Geographies 2002; 9: 467–71.

Brown J. ARTnode audio guide. (CD). University of Newcastle, NSW, Australia: John Gray, 2003.

Hankinson C. The Experience and Effect of Creative Activities for Participants in a Community Arts Project. University of Newcastle, NSW, Australia, unpublished manuscript, 2002.

Material Women: weaving fabric and stories

Perth, Australia

Margaret Ross and Katie Hill

Margaret and Katie were two occupational therapists with a passion for promoting health and wellness through active participation in valued occupations or activities. In addition, they had a deep concern about the visibility of women's stories, and recognition of their contribution to their families and communities, so they became involved in the absorbing project called 'Material Women '99'. This was one of the projects celebrating 100 years of women's suffrage in Western Australia in 1999. The project used storytelling, and the depiction of these stories on quilts, as a way to acknowledge the achievements of women (Hill and Ross, 1999). Brief mention is also made of a subsequent project, 'Connecting Arts', which was inspired by the success of quilting as creative storytelling and shared activity.

This is a report, compiled in November 2003, by Margaret Ross with contributions from Katie Hill. Margaret now works part-time as a research consultant and golfer in Albany. Katie works full-time at the WA Network and WA Guardianship Board in Perth.

'Material Women '99'

This project began in late 1996 when the two of us (Margaret and Katie) began to have regular informal meetings about graduate studies, and, invariably, our conversation would cover the importance of using personal experiences in order to move forward in life. We felt women's life stories were frequently viewed as trivial, or were invisible. Margaret was writing her doctoral thesis on the career stories of women managers in health services, and found this state of invisibility to be a recurring issue. As it was around the time preparations were being made to celebrate the centenary of women's suffrage in Western Australia, we two friends came to an agreement that quilts could be a creative and colourful way to tell stories and promote women's issues. We received a small grant from the state government, and Katie became the project co-ordinator. We talked to everyone who would listen to our ideas, presented a workshop at the 'Women in Leadership' conference, and because neither of us were experienced quilters we established contact with the WA Quilters' Association.

Katie focused on developing an exhibition of quilts, each one depicting and celebrating the life of a Western Australian woman. The invitation was extended to anyone who was willing to make a quilt and write about the person's contribution to her family or community. Sixty-six quilts, of varying sizes, were created by individuals and groups with a range of experiences, of all ages, and from across the city and countryside. One of the most exciting days of my professional life happened when the quilts were handed in to us for the exhibition. It was time for the preparation of the publication showing the quilts beside the story. There was considerable excitement and pride as the makers and storytellers presented their quilts.

Some of these comments from participants convey their variety of experiences, plus their enthusiasm and enjoyment in this creative occupation:

> 'When I first heard about the quilting project I had no experience with patchwork or quilting, but I decided it was a brilliant idea, as I appreciate women having the vote. I started quilting classes, and became enthusiastic about the whole concept. I have really enjoyed this project, and the family have thought it was great too.' (Betty)

In contrast to Betty, who worked alone on her first quilt, Lynette was an experienced quilter:

> 'I began quilting around 15 years ago when I joined a local group. We meet every Monday afternoon and have formed strong friendships, making quilts as a group for one another's birthdays (60 is the magic year), and also for charitable institutions. I have entered exhibitions and shows regularly over the years. (Lynette)

Some participants used 'Material Women '99' to celebrate their family traditions, whereas others used this project to pay tribute to a famous community achiever, Dr Fiona Stanley.

> 'I made a quilt representing our district, and my grandmother made an ideal subject. The story was written by my aunt with the help of many family members, and fellow patch workers have provided encouragement, ideas and a helping hand.' (Judy)

> 'I work with support staff in different health facilities. This project has been a wonderful opportunity for us to get together and to pool our creative skills, as well as contribute to a community project.' (Pat)

Many quilters talked about the positive benefits of being involved in this creative project and the social connections they made that provided support through difficult times:

> 'Patchwork quilting is of recent interest and is now my relaxation.' (Gail)

> 'I began quilting in 1983, and through quilting I have acquired many friends who helped me tremendously after losing our youngest son in January this year. Being part of this project has been a life saver – and my aunt is thrilled to be my subject as she is now 92 years old.' (Val)

> '. . . part of the team, with Elsje the leader – guiding, inspiring and setting the pace. So our lives touched as we worked ever harder, enjoying the challenge, which seemed like a race. We all were winners, this band of achievers, dispersed now but changed by the bond never broken. Regrouped and reformed, we dyed, cut and sewed our homage to Elsje, who inspired this our token.' (Jill)

Elsje was their textile lecturer, and she had taken her students on bush camps to learn about dyeing and creative use of fabrics, and the inspiration of nature, while also learning about themselves. This group used silk and dyed their sections of material before joining together as a group to create their piece of fabric. This was a wonderful tribute to the contribution Elsje had made to their lives, personal development and creativity.

These comments and the pictures of the quilts remind me of the joy and satisfaction we all felt when the 'Material Women '99' exhibition was opened and the book was launched. The quilt exhibition toured the state and inspired many people to value women's contribution to society. Some years later I am still talking about the benefits and positive outcomes of this creative project. The project still resonates strongly with women, quilters, storytellers and the community. The extra piece to this project is the research evaluation we conducted to investigate the link between this leisure occupation and health. From all these anecdotal comments we wanted some evidence that quilting was a meaningful occupation that promoted health and well-being.

Research project: the occupation of quilting

This research project investigated the relationship between a leisure occupation and health. The purpose of the research was to develop an understanding of the occupation of quilting, and to explore the way that women include quilting as part of a life of meaningful occupation. The study also explored the potential of quilting as a means of promoting health and well-being. The domain of occupational science provided the theoretical foundation for the research. Occupational science is grounded in the concept that people are occupational beings, and that on a day-to-day basis, occupations are used as the basis for quality of life, wellness, empowerment and social equity.

The research design for the study used both qualitative (interview transcripts and participant observation) and quantitative methods (210 questionnaires distributed to city and country areas). After detailed statistical and thematic analysis, the findings were grouped into the following parts:

- the characteristics of women who see themselves as quilters
- the reasons why women quilt
- the selection of quilting as a preferred leisure occupation
- the dimensions of the occupation and benefits of quilting.

Engaging in quilting appears to be important for two reasons: personal pleasure experienced during the creative process and the opportunity to form strong social connections and share with others. The implications from this research cover both the practice of occupational therapy and the demonstration of a process to study many other occupations. The design process and making a meaningful product provided satisfaction and purpose to everyday activities, which then contributed to strengthening the women's occupational identity. In addition, the evidence of the strong social benefits and emotional connections made through this creative occupation suggests that therapists could make more links with community groups to provide support for isolated, depressed and at-risk groups. Participants described how social support had a buffering effect when coping with stresses, and gave them resilience through their sense of connectedness and attachment to networks within the community. They said that this productive, creative task gave them meaning and purpose in life. Involvement in groups provided pleasurable experiences and laughter that had a positive effect on their feelings and mood. The occupation of quilting provided a challenging and rewarding creative outlet as well as a sense of satisfaction and self-worth. Several research participants stated:

'I am happiest when quilting which must help my sense of well-being.'

'You have to struggle to develop skills and abilities but you get a real buzz when you have met a challenge and finished a quilt.'

'the company of others and the enjoyment of creating something is important to one's well-being.'

'I love the sense of achievement and satisfaction, the opportunity to be creative when working with fabric and great colours.'

The findings of our study supported the initial expectation that women engage in quilting because they know it provides pleasure, makes them feel good and creates a sense of satisfaction, fulfilment and pride. It provides opportunity to be creative, and some women found it to be therapeutic and relaxing. The outcome of quilting, that is, the finished item, is a visible and lasting proof of achievement. The importance of this creative activity is also related to the social component. Participants wrote about getting ideas from others, swapping fabric, mutual support, enjoying laughter and having a glass of wine together. Company and friendship were clearly an integral part of the process. We believe that quilters are a fortunate group of people who have chosen a valued leisure time occupation that provides a supportive circle of friends, and allows for the production of creative and highly treasured outcomes. Also, it provides active and meaningful engagement in a personal passion that provides a sense of achievement in their everyday life.

'Connecting Arts': celebrating reconciliation and renewal

Again, having experienced the power of creative arts, I applied for funding for a reconciliation project, 'Connecting Arts', at Curtin University, for staff and students. In this second project we used playback theatre, storytelling and a range of expressive media including art, quilting and pottery. The groups used these media to develop themes of understanding, tolerance and harmony, as well as to acknowledge the positive images of diversity. The outcomes of this project are displayed on the walls of the university and provided the basis of an experiential workshop at an international action research conference.

Conclusion

You can see from these absorbing projects, 'Material Women '99' and 'Connecting Arts', that Katie and I became more enthusiastic about our chosen profession and the opportunities to be involved in creative projects and work with community groups. We have enjoyed the challenges and problem-solving, adding further to our friendship and support of each other through domestic and work-related crises, and sharing much laughter along the way:

> Together we planted the seed of an idea, an exhibition of quilts in celebration of the centenary of women's suffrage in Western Australia. Together we watered, mulched, hoed and pruned until we were able to gather the fruits. We both value our ability to work as a team. (Hill and Ross, 1999, p. 112)

We are all authors of our own life stories. We have the choice of occupations and activities with which to create ourselves – our identities as occupational beings.

Reference

Hill K, Ross M. Material Women '99: Quilts That Tell Stories. Perth, Western Australia: Curtin University of Technology, 1999.

Acknowledgements

Centenary of Women's Suffrage Committee, Women's Policy Office, Government of Western Australia, Australian Association of Occupational Therapists WA (Inc) Research Grant, Occupational Therapists Registration Board of Western Australia Research Grant, Curtin University of Technology Vice Chancellor's Discretionary Reserve Fund, and participants of all these projects.

Further information, references and resources

Pendleton HH. The occupation of needlework. In: Zemke R, Clarke F (eds). Occupational Science: The Evolving Discipline. Philadelphia, PA: FA Davis, 1996; 287–95.

'Friendship Quilts, 2003'. Suzanne Nield, a grazier from south-western NSW, Australia, came up with an idea to help communities suffering the depressions of drought. Her aim was to bring women together to do something worthwhile, enjoyable, and to get away from everyday problems. This was not a funded project. Suzanne arranged social days, including quilting workshops, where women met together to produce quilts. The women produced some 150 quilts, are planning to hold an exhibition and auction the quilts for charity. When discussing her experiences of this project, Suzanne spoke about the positive social connections the women experienced. She spoke of how the women networked with others whom they thought were isolated and involved them in the project, and of the changes she observed in the women's self-confidence. Suzanne also said that after the project was finished, the women were 'wanting to keep going, organizing other craft days'. In response to the discussion on the effect that the activity had on people's health and well-being, Suzanne summed it up by saying: 'Creativity gives us a healthy mind' (S. Nield, personal communication, October 22, 2003).

'Textile Fibre Forum', NSW, Australia has been going for 30 years and holds forum workshops and conferences. 'Camp Creative', in NSW, Australia offers creative activities and skill-building workshops for children and families. These groups hold the promise of revealing the connection between creativity and health and well-being.

Development of Creativity: an alternative path to health

Department of Education in Health Sciences, Faculty of Medicine, University of Chile

Dr Ximena Gonzalez

I have been working for many years with pre-graduate students, trying to help them to discover and develop their creative potential. I have also worked with professional people (from areas such as education, arts, health, sciences, social sciences, etc.) on the same issue, through postgraduate courses at the Faculty of Medicine and other faculties and universities. The objectives are to find the barriers that have inhibited their creativity, to develop creative factors of personality, to discover different ways to face problems and to solve them, but especially, to be able to ask new questions and find new points of view.

For me, one of the most attractive abilities of the human being is the capacity for dreaming, in the most ample meaning of the word: to dream a better world; to ask yourself questions; not to accept things as they 'are'; to ask yourself if there is some other way.

I tell people to ask themselves, 'Who said I couldn't?' It is a very disquieting question. You discover you were doing a lot of things, believing that you had to do them, and in just one way of doing them. Why?

I tell them that it is quite a subversive question: you will have to redefine all your beliefs; you will have to choose your opinions, your values, your principles, your behaviour, your way of relating with other people and with nature; your way of expressing your feelings; and your own way to belong.

All this means hard work. You will have to explore your mind and your soul. You will have to fight with the world that is trying to tell you to conform to its rules. You will have to create a whole new set of values, principles and behaviours, but they will have to be dynamic and flexible. It is a whole life work; you will have to be alert all the time, or you will slide again to the common state of belonging to the herd . . . it is so much easier!

We work in groups, using expressive activities (corporal work, dance, drawing, painting, writing, dramatizations, singing, masks, etc.), psychodrama and specific creativity techniques. One of the most important themes is to create a feeling of acceptance and belonging in the group. It is achieved through the playful characteristic of the workshop and the facilitating attitude of the co-ordinator. At the end of the first session, people are already at ease.

This workshop has a predetermined duration of at least 12 three-hour sessions, depending on the objectives and the participants (the postgraduate course has a duration of one year of two academic semesters). Each session has a specific objective (for instance, to discover emotional barriers). At the end of each session there is a time to share feelings and to search the theoretical concepts of the work done. Participants relate their changes in a self-evaluation form at the end of the workshop. There are also different evaluations during the course (portfolio, practice, group presentations of a theme, a final 'group performance').

One of the most interesting things that appear in these evaluations is the feeling of deep changes in participants' mental health. Even though the workshops and courses have an 'academic' objective, people tend to value more their emotional achievements, the sense of well-being, the happiness of being able to do different things, the possibility of destroying obstacles that were inhibiting their development as individuals, the ability to have better relationships, to be able to express their feelings in adequate ways, the gaining of self-esteem, a feeling of connection and of 'opening the doors of perception'.

Many participants have told me that they feel their life has changed, that there is a 'before and after the workshop'. They relate this change to a deep understanding of the values and principles that underlie all the workshops. It is not only learning new techniques or concepts; it is a different way of connecting with themselves and with the world. These are some comments from pre-graduate occupational therapy students:

'It helped me very much, because I realized how I am and why I have these barriers in my mind.'

'This course teaches us to look at things in a different way. It is easier for me to do things that I have never done before. I am less critical; accepting of other people's opinions. I can share my feelings and ideas in a better way.'

'It has helped me a lot, I have used many things I learnt here, in my everyday life.'

'I feel less blockaded. I think that now I am more frank, more sincere.'

'I have learnt to be more flexible. I can be more objective in front of problems.'

'Before, I would clam like an oyster, nobody would be able to make me think in a different way.'

'It allowed me to find and affirm my creative potential.'

'I believe now I have less obstacles.'

'Now I have more skills – some I did have and didn't know I had – creativity skills that I can use in all fields of my life.'

'I have noticed changes. At first I didn't dare to do some things. Now I feel that I have more personality.'

'It helped me to understand that we have a potentiality that is hidden, something very deep, that is waiting to come to the outside. It is excellent for self-esteem.'

'I could recognize some negative aspects of my personality and change them.'

'We are a better group now, we feel the acceptance, based in a deep confidence among us. We have a strong affective link among us.'

'Now I can find different answers for problems.'

People that have participated in the post-graduate courses tell me about how this experience has stayed with them, the feeling of inner freedom, of mental and physical health, of being able to make difficult decisions without fear, of facing risks knowing they have the ability to find their own path, and the capacity to work in creative teams. Also, that they are able to transmit these achievements to other people. Many of them are applying the issues learnt at the course in their professions, especially in teaching and in health promotion.

Further information

See also Chapter 8 in this book.
Schmid T. Experiential art exercises as learning tools in teaching communication. Teaching Review 1996; December: 12–16.

Summary and conclusion

All the group projects described in this chapter provided creative activity as a service to people who were healthy or to those who were in recovery from an illness or had a disability, or those who were marginalized; that is, youth, the elderly or those with an enduring illness. All of the projects had, as an aim, an outcome of increased health and well-being. This is described in many different ways, for example, as an increase in social connection (refer to the term 'social health', in Chapter 1), or as individual and community health in the form of increased self-esteem or self-confidence. This chapter aimed to describe the value these projects had for participants' health and well-being, and to stimulate readers to perceive opportunities for research. What is obvious, as in Chapter Seven, is that all of the accounts do, in one way or another, express a highly valued involvement in creative activities, and all demonstrate a belief that benefits are to be obtained from that involvement. Evaluations were discussed in the contributions from the 'Older People's Circus' and the 'Development of Creativity'. 'The Wilderness Theatre', the 'Material Women: weaving fabric and stories', and the 'Sculpture Trail: ARTnode' described research undertaken. These projects provided a glimpse of the kind of design methodology that could be applied to like projects.

CHAPTER 10

What is to be done?

THERESE SCHMID

What is creativity for health and well-being? A summary

So far we have examined the available research and experience that sub-stantiates the argument that creativity is beneficial to health and well-being. This research reveals the innate creative capacity that every person could benefit from, if only they could be encouraged to take advantage of it. The review of the complex concepts of the phenomena of creativity and health has resulted in the new definition of creativity, which appears in Chapters One and Two.

The notion that creativity can be a major part of everyday activities was introduced and grounded within the occupational theory of human nature, and in the notions of occupational genesis through our knowl-edge of human evolution and the extraordinary biological changes that have enabled the creative capacities that are innate in everybody. These notions offer a significant theoretical framework for the link between cre-ativity and health and well-being, and for further creativity research.

The evidence drawn from neuroscience, psychology and education of the 'affective states' (the feelings of pleasure, happiness, achievement, excite-ment, to name a few) being an outcome of creativity, further validates the new definition of creativity. Reynolds, in summarizing new directions for research in Chapter Five, suggested that further studies are needed, especially those that are self-reporting and use phenomenological research methods to reveal people's subjective experience of the creative process. This kind of research has been missing and, when used, it will be complementary to the bulk of quantitative research used at present. Chapters Seven and Nine have revealed the significance of the notions about the affective states to this emerging field. The individual and group accounts were designed to offer rich subjective nar-ratives, which link creativity to health and well-being, and to stimulate ideas for research using qualitative methodologies.

The material in Denshire's Chapter Eight described the astonishing positive effects on participants' health and well-being of combining creativity and groupwork. This supports the outcomes of the group and project experiences described in Chapter Nine. The other consistent and convincing evidence of the benefits of creativity for health and well-being has come from long years of clinical therapeutic practice by clinicians, and has been described by Creek in Chapter Four.

The preceding chapters have offered a rich panorama of agreements about a vast field of study that is wide open for adventurous researchers. The book supports the 'promotion of the abundant life', a view which is held by the Honourable Dr Barry Jones, AO, who also stated 'the overwhelming majority of people are capable of responding to a far greater richness of experience than is commonly recognised' (Labor Herald, 2000). Creativity, with its many facets, is a growing field of study. A groundswell of interest exists, and new courses involving arts and health professionals have been created as a result. This book, in part, aims to encourage those prospective students and researchers by providing theoretical perspectives which can underlie practice and research.

Many people to whom I have spoken about this book have expressed surprise that it is needed. However, when looking at the literature and the health in the community, the response to this is obvious. Not enough is written about the significance of creativity. Our society does not explicate it or support it on the same level as the issues of exercise and healthy diet, yet the biological connection is present.

Why is this an issue now?

The effects of rapid changes in our technological society remain unabated. Jones (1995) aptly described the causes as follows:

> The Western world is passing through a period of technological change more far-reaching and much faster than at any other time. This rapidity and intensity presents massive challenges. The technicalities are easy to solve: The human problems of understanding complex and shifting technological matters and assessing their social impact are more difficult. (Jones, 1995, pp 259–60).

These effects have been addressed by many writers and are discussed in Chapters Two and Three. Jones (1995, p. 261) called us to question, 'are we well enough equipped to make sensible collective and individual decisions about our futures?' Jones offered solutions for policy as well as for individuals and communities, to help us raise our levels of consciousness if we are 'to get the best and not the worst out of the coming changes –

to play active life-enhancing roles . . . will make a major contribution to mental health' (Jones, 1995, p. 256).

The statistics are warning us of an epidemic of mental health problems (refer to Chapter 1). Is the epidemic a result of the rapid changes? It looks very likely. Promoting *creativity for health and well-being* as a life skill could make a major contribution to providing an aid for positive mental health. With all the changes and disruptions in society, creativity is a great resource for maintaining self-esteem. That is why it is necessary to provide policymakers in health, education and arts with good evidence and reasons to devise policies, using creativity, to provide resources to minimize mental health problems and consequent ill-health.

Furthermore, as discussed in Chapter Two, there are many layers of sociocultural values that hide the reality of creativity in everyday activities, and these layers must be peeled back to reveal that there are important choices to be made about whether to utilize our capacities for creativity.

Creativity in education is not new. A wealth of literature exists which describes theories, research, and a myriad of successful methods for practice involving creativity. Many authors, including Rogers (1954; as cited in Vernon, 1970), Read (1964), Kneller (1965), Barron (1969), Maslow (1971), Edwards (1986), Isaksen et al. (1993), Torrance (1995) and Cropley (1997, 1999), have, for decades, advocated the promotion of creativity in education. However, the notion that creativity is a biological need is not explicated widely. Keeping in tune with our biological needs is an important part of keeping us healthy as a species (Wilcock, 1998). This book has aimed to advance the notion that creativity can be a part of everyday activities and is an innate capacity and therefore linked to health and well-being. What prevents people from understanding and accepting creativity for its healthful role in everyday activities is that they are not aware of health's dependence on the biological capacities.

The book describes an emerging field of practice and research for a wide range of health and arts health professionals and educationalists. It provides an integration of multidisciplinary literature and offers suggestions that could contribute to a common language. Distinguished creativity researchers Robert Sternberg, Department of Psychology at Yale University, Mark Runco, editor of the prestigious journal *Creativity Research* and Scott Isaksen and co-authors (1993) in their book, *Nurturing and Developing Creativity*, have been calling for new perspectives from their own field and from multidisciplinary fields of research. This book has responded to their challenge.

Psychologists such as Guilford (1950) and subsequent creativity researchers have written and researched this area for 50 years. However, the research methodologies have been limited, for they have focused on small components of a big picture. Of course, this research has been incredibly valuable. It has given huge insights into the workings of creativity. But what has been lacking is the 'big picture': the effect of the innate creative capacity on health and well-being, which is within the realm of qualitative research methodologies. This book brings the 'big picture' into focus.

What is to be done?

The effects of rapid changes are so challenging that it seems new approaches and partnerships need to be established in order to address these serious issues. The following suggestions are made. The issue in this book is for us to not neglect creativity as a useful resource. It urges the adoption of new approaches and long-term strategies. It urges public health to embrace creativity within their fields of research, promotion and practice, and to include creative needs within the population healthcare model. It urges that partnerships be formed between all health, arts and education departments, and organizations in order to recognize, plan and exploit the resource effectively. A new image of creativity must be generated so that it can be understood that our natural capacity for creativity can be readily expressed in healthy balanced everyday activities and occupations, and so that it can be recognized as not only rewarding and pleasurable, but also as biologically essential to our health and well-being.

Leadership at all levels is a likely place to commence. Leaders will readily recognize that their achievements arise from the combination of their skills and their creative capabilities. Leadership, therefore, could set the example openly. Government planners and their operational structures could be encouraged to promote the kinds of creative activities within occupations, recreation and daily living that contribute to a healthy life.

Long-term strategies

Jones (1995) recommended long-term strategies to address the effects of rapid change. Policymakers and politicians are in the ideal position to promote the various health determinants and to recognize that the problem of denied creativity is immense. The worst thing that could happen is that we do nothing:

> Many people feel reluctant to face up to the issues and would prefer to put off thinking about them in the hope that either the problems will go away or prove to be exaggerated, or someone else might solve them (or take the blame if they propose solutions which then prove to be wrong – or unpopular). (Jones, 1995, pp 259–60)

A long-term goal would be to create or revive the perception that it is good and positive to integrate creativity, as an innate human capacity and need, with everyday activities because the outcomes are positive for health and well-being. One hurdle to overcome is the confusion over the concepts of health, ill-health, mental health and well-being, health promotion and illness prevention (*see* Chapter 1). A consensus of what meaning is intended with these words could set a policy for a common language that could be widely accepted. Long-term strategies would include those for healthy individuals and healthy populations, as well as for individuals with ill-health and unhealthy populations.

Long-term strategies are required because so many layers of sociocultural perceptions, values and beliefs have suppressed creativity. For many it has become the accepted thing that they are not creative or that creativity is not needed. They have learnt that everything they need is available to them through the creative efforts of others. It takes energy to think, to problem-solve, to invent and to innovate. The easy way out will do; life will be good anyway. Many people have not learnt to experience the pleasure of the outcomes of creativity. In fact, in many cases they have not been taught about the processes of creativity and do not know what they are missing. They have learnt, however, that creativity seems to be the realm of the artists, the sculptors, the musicians and the dancers. That seems remote and unattainable, and not even desirable, so why try! But occasionally they solve a problem and feel good about it. They may not recognize it as creativity, but it is. That same rewarding experience can become bigger and better and more frequent, and those good feelings are the origins of self-esteem, and self-esteem is the basis of well-being. Within this little story are a host of barriers that will have to be broken down. The long-term key for that is through education, and through learning how creativity really functions and how to make it work at will.

We can make a difference by providing people with the opportunity to be creative. It does not seem enough to leave it to individuals to be aware that their health can benefit from creativity. The solution is in education. Teaching about creativity must not be confused with teaching about the arts. The latter is already available. The subject for education here is the nature and practice of the processes of creativity so that they may be applied in all or any activities throughout life, including the arts. If it can become commonplace in education, at all levels, for creativity to be a conscious tool, without self-consciousness, then it may become a part of all everyday activities. The benefits are potentially enormous for the enjoyment of life, the growth of self-esteem and the maintenance of health. The incidence of depression could be reduced. The community's very large financial health burden could be significantly reduced. In the long term the financial costs of the whole programme would be more than offset by the gains.

To achieve all this, the new processes of education, community activity and opportunity, starting with health education, would require significant funding. For example, there would be the need for all teachers to be taught, and there would be the need to establish centres of excellence, specializing in creativity research and teaching. The learning process would continue throughout all education, thus becoming a lifetime activity. Creativity would therefore be promoted in all areas of occupations and professions in such a way that it is valued as a productive skill. Concurrently, the rewards of creativity in terms of achievement, satisfaction and health, and well-being would have to be promoted in the community.

'Creative Connections' (VicHealth, 2002) showcases a variety of cutting-edge projects which promote health, mental well-being and social and community well-being through arts activities. To take this work further, it is suggested that the *population healthcare* model could be used as a framework for future projects that incorporate creativity in everyday activities across the whole population. The *universal preventive intervention* level of the population healthcare model would be a valuable level at which the promotion of health and well-being through creativity could take place. Various education methods could be designed, ranging from media campaigns to education systems at all levels. The designs for the promotion of these notions could be similar to those used for the promotion of exercise and healthy diet.

Funding more community *early intervention* services, through a population healthcare model, that provide a range of creative activities could offer increased opportunities for those people who are depressed, low in confidence and self-esteem, and for the vulnerable, healthy aged.

Current community *selective and indicated mental illness prevention intervention* (population healthcare model) and the *mental illness treatment and maintenance services* within psychiatric settings do not provide, as yet, a sufficient range of creative activities for their clients. Some settings do provide a creative arts programme and these are important examples of what could be multiplied in many different ways and at many different levels (refer to the example of VICSERV in Chapter 9).

Long-term funding could be considered. Too few projects have enjoyed sustained funding. Some exceptions are Artsenta in New Zealand, Sound Minds in the UK and Artful Dodger in Australia, all of which were described in Chapter Nine. Funding long-term projects would, in part, enable substantial research to prove and define successful programme styles, and enable the testing of new research designs and methodologies.

Changes in beliefs and perceptions: some promotional directions

Recognizing the value of creativity and activating it within our daily life as individuals and as communities is a way of getting the best out of the difficult changes and disruptions in our modern society. Novel, personally developed strategies play a vital role in enhancing the quality of everyday life. With a creative background, every individual should be part of solving that problem. Sitting back and waiting for life to deal a good card is wishful thinking without any likely outcome. Awareness of the values that creativity can bring to health, well-being and quality of life must be cultivated. Changes in beliefs, values and perception are very difficult to make. This book is urging for creativity to be reinvented. It could be difficult but it is not impossible. Serious and successful campaigns have already been organized in Australia warning about the AIDS epidemic and the dangers of smoking.

The following points are suggested as the bases for the promotion of 'creativity for health and well-being':

- Creativity, in the forms of problem solving, ingenuity, innovation and inventiveness, is an innate capacity of everyone, that can be exercised at will and can be applied to everyday activities.
- The positive feelings elicited by creativity – feelings of pleasure, excitement, satisfaction (*see* Chapter 2) should be described as an outcome and component of creativity that can be a vital part of positive health and well-being.
- Creativity is as vital to health and well-being as are physical exercise and diet.
- Creativity does not just belong to people involved in the arts. It is a useful, practical and exciting tool to be used for all manner of ventures. Creativity derives from our survival skills, and it is still that if it can give us quality of life.
- Creativity can be used in many situations. It can be used to solve all kinds of problems. It can be used for devising all kinds of aids or artefacts. It can be used to create something beautiful. It can be a distracter from painful and negative thoughts. It can help prevent and alleviate some types of depression. It can sometimes even be used to achieve the apparently impossible.
- Our creativity is valuable, and we should cultivate it and call upon it at every opportunity.
- Creative activity within groups of like-minded people will provide a positive sense of social belonging. The creative input of others is valuable. We should value it, assess it and utilize it, if it has the potential to

add value of any kind. This can enable us to help each other to cultivate the skills of accessing and using our creativity.
- Talking about creativity intelligently without being coy or self-
conscious is very important and demands a little time devoted to learning the language of creativity.
- The differences between the concepts of health promotion and illness prevention should be understood, that is, from the point of view of what
constitutes a healthy life rather than the absence of disease (*see* Chapter 1).
- The definition of health should incorporate an occupational perspective.
It is vital to the health of a nation for everyone to know what are healthy
activities and what are unhealthy activities. Healthy occupation is a
requirement for healthy living (Wilcock, 1998); people need meaningful
and purposeful activities in order to experience health and well-being.

While promoting creativity for positive health and well-being, it may also
be useful to articulate what creativity is not (van Kaam, 1966; Streubert
and Carpenter, 1995). Creativity is a vital part of the arts, but it is not
defined by or limited to the arts. Creativity is not something that belongs
only to the élite and talented. Similarly, creativity is not 'therapy', 'art therapy' or 'crafts', although it can be utilized in all three.

Forming partnerships

The following suggestions may be useful for partnership activities.

- Policy and funding partnerships between public health, health-
promotion, education and various arts organizations could be undertaken at all levels. Long-range strategies would be required to facilitate
new perceptions and services. A 'big picture' view should be considered for the funding of all of the co-operating bodies.
- Multidisciplinary partnerships with health, arts and education would
be important for creativity research and learning centres, in substanti-
ating and validating new directions. (*See* the next section, 'Centres for
creativity research'.)
- Establishing creative arts programmes can empower communities. A
recent example of pioneering collaboration and partnership was
formed between the Cultural Development Network of Victoria,
Australia, and the Centre for Sustainable Regional Communities at La
Trobe University in Bendigo, Victoria, Australia. This project, 'Small
Towns, Big Picture', was described in Chapter Nine. A sophisticated
programme of creative-arts activities was developed with the aim of
empowering several communities. It was very successful and positively
benefited the health and well-being of all of the communities involved.

- Teachers could consider establishing partnerships. The arts as creative activities are vehicles (although not the only ones) used for teaching the creative process, and are effective for teaching the creative skills that can be applied in everyday activities. However, is this the domain of all teachers, or of only speciality teachers? Teachers could collaborate to form a programme for explicating the creative process and how this can be applied to everyday activities in the form of problem finding, problem-solving and innovating in practical matters, in self-direction, in relationships, in learning processes and in balancing life-style with meaningful and purposeful activities, all with the bonus of self-esteem that promotes health and well-being.

Centres for creativity research

Establishing centres for research and studies in creativity within universities could validate and assist the process of this proposed new education, new community activity and new opportunity. Universities could champion the notions of creativity for health and well-being by explicating them within existing academic courses and by offering learning for external students. Establishing partnerships with health, arts and education could provide excellent wide-ranging opportunities for research and deliver quality guidance in the application of the knowledge gained.

The centres could facilitate postgraduate research and a variety of learning programmes and courses. For example, postgraduate programmes could be offered in creativity for health and well-being, community health through the arts, creative arts therapies, and innovation. In addition, the following short courses, workshops and seminars could be offered: creativity for health professionals; creativity in therapy; creativity in management; creativity in business; creativity in leadership; creative comprehension; arts-in-health; and creative problem-solving for many fields, including health, education, arts, commerce, industry and community development.

Funding for innovative postgraduate courses in this field should be considered. A wide variety of health and arts health professionals are already requiring further knowledge and practice in this area. The number of postgraduate arts courses in music, dance and movement therapy, art therapy and drama therapy has increased significantly, as is described in Chapter One.

Some recommended research projects

New directions for research into creativity-related topics have been suggested in chapters Five and Six. The topics identified are current issues and seem to be a priority for immediate research. One example of these suggestions is for research based on women's and men's own narrative accounts of growing up in families and schools that nurtured or inhibited creativity, and of the subsequent impact on their lives. A second suggestion is for research based on the use of case studies and biographies of certain acclaimed artists who have been spurred into art through illness or injury. Reynolds, in Chapter 5, explained:

> Such confinement to home (and in many cases to bed) resulted in the experience of unproductive time and the search for a meaningful activity. Illness also confronts the sufferer with issues around self, anxiety and mortality. Some individuals appear to address these deeper concerns through creative self-expression.

It is such a pity that it should take such a crisis to bring out a realization of one's creativity capacity and the desire to use it, rather than have it understood from a young age.

Creativity should not be the province of the fortunate few. The distinguishing personality and cognitive attributes that acclaimed creative people have from an early age implies a need for better nurturance of children's creative potential within the educational system. This is indeed a topic for further research.

It is recommended that research be carried out to compare the benefits gained from individual creative activity and the benefits gained from creative activity in groups. As Denshire has discussed in Chapter Eight, drawing on van Gennep (1960), Kitzinger (1977) and Mahdi et al. (1987), 'Group participation provides peers and mutual support . . . The current lack of rituals in society may leave people with a hunger that could be satisfied through meaningful creativity-based group participation.'

The problem of rural and remote youth who are at risk of depression and suicide has been identified in public-health policy as a major target for mental-health promotion and education. Denshire, in Chapter Eight, has discussed at length the benefits accruing to youth who engage in creative group activity. It is suggested that community mental health promotion and education for such rural and remote youth include more creative activity programmes. If participants were given opportunities to see creativity as a skill in everyday activities, they would be informed to make a choice about accepting this as something that can be learnt, enjoyed and applied to increasing self-esteem and coping skills. Research is needed to assess such programmes and how they might encourage novel, personally developed strategies to improve the quality of everyday life.

Final notes

Creativity adds that little bit of difference to a task or an activity. It is the spice, the pepper, the icing on the cake. It is an ingredient. It is not the preparation or the cooking of the food, for this is the skill. Many artists and highly expressive creative people have worked very hard and long at developing their skills in specific areas. However, it is the adding of that special creativity, that special ingredient, which makes them distinctive. Training in creativity is enormously worthwhile, for it has incredible spin-offs for problem solving and innovation.

In the light of the increasing incidence of mental health problems, in particular depression, we now need to make use of all the resources and strategies available in order to survive psychologically. The creative capacity could enable people to optimize their resources and strategies. If governments embraced and financially supported these educative notions, the value of creativity would be generally recognized and accepted, and then we would see developing an exciting environment for health improvement.

Doing something new about creativity as a resource is an economic need. That is clear from the growing burden of health costs. The human need to alleviate and avoid ill-health is even greater. If creativity, as a resource, is accepted, the chances for a satisfying occupation and rewarding lifestyle will be enhanced and the risk of mental disturbances will be diminished.

References

Barron F. Creative Person and Creative Process. New York, NY: Holt, Rinehart & Winston, 1969.

Cropley AJ. Fostering creativity in the classroom: general principles. In: Runco MA (ed.), The Creativity Handbook. Cresskill, NJ: Hampton Press, 1997; 83–114.

Cropley AJ. Education. In: Runco MA, Pritzker SR (eds), Encyclopedia of Creativity (Vol. 1). London: Academic Press, 1999; 629–37.

Edwards B. Drawing on the Artist Within. How to Release your Hidden Creativity. Glasgow: Fontana/Collins, 1986.

van Gennep A. The Rites of Passage (trans. MB Vizedom, GL Caffee). Chicago, IL: University of Chicago, 1960.

Guilford JP. Creativity. American Psychologist 1950; 5: 444–54.

Isaksen SG, Murdock MC, Firestien RL, Treffinger DJ. Nurturing and Developing Creativity: The Emergence of a Discipline. Norwood, NJ: Ablex, 1993.

Jones B. Sleepers, Wake! Technology and the Future of Work (fourth edition). Melbourne, Victoria, Australia: Oxford University Press, 1995.

van Kaam A. Existential Foundations of Psychology. Garden City, NY: Image, 1966.

Kitzinger S. Education and Counselling for Childbirth. London: Cassell & Collier Macmillan, 1977.

Kneller GF. The Art and Science of Creativity. New York, NY: Holt, Reinhart & Winston, 1965.

Labor Herald. Always looking forward – Barry Jones. October 2000. (Accessed 1 July 2004: www.alp.org.au/laborherald/october2000/ jones.html)

Mahdi LC, Foster S, Little M (eds). Betwixt and Between: Patterns of Masculine and Feminine Initiation. La Salle, IL: Open Court, 1987.

Maslow AH. The Farther Reaches of Human Nature. New York, NY: Viking, 1971.

Read H. Art and Education. Melbourne, Victoria, Australia: FW Cheshire, 1964.

Streubert HJ, Carpenter DR. Qualitative Research in Nursing. Philadelphia, PA: JB Lippincott, 1995.

Torrance EP. Why Fly? A Philosophy of Creativity. Norwood, NJ: Ablex, 1995.

Vernon PE. Creativity. Selected Readings. New York, NY: Penguin Books, 1970.

VicHealth. Creative Connections: Promoting Mental Health and Well-being through Community Arts Participation. Melbourne, Victoria, Australia: Victoria Health Promotion Foundation, 2002.

Wilcock AA. An Occupational Perspective of Health. Thorofare, NJ: Slack, 1998.

Index